A Veterinary Practitioner Handbook
Series Edited by Neal King BVSC MRCVS

NOTES ON CANINE
INTERNAL MEDICINE

P. G. G. Darke BVSc, PhD, MRCVS, DVR

Director, Small Animal Clinic,
University of Edinburgh

Second Edition

WRIGHT
Bristol
1986

Published
under the Wright Imprint by IOP Publishing Limited,
Techno House, Redcliffe Way, Bristol BS1 6NX

First edition, 1983
Second edition, 1986

British Library Cataloguing in Publication Data

Darke, P. G. G.
    Notes on canine internal medicine.—
    2nd ed.—(A veterinary practitioner handbook)
    1.   Dogs—Diseases
    I.   Title   II. Series
    636.7′0896   SF991

ISBN 0 7236 0887 3

Typeset by
Severntype Repro Services Ltd,
Market Street, Wotton-under-Edge, Glos.

Printed in Great Britain by
Billing and Sons Ltd, Worcester

A Veterinary Practitioner Handbook
Series Edited by Neal King BVSC MRCVS

NOTES ON CANINE INTERNAL MEDICINE

P. G. G. Darke BVSc, PhD, MRCVS, DVR

Director, Small Animal Clinic,
University of Edinburgh

Second Edition

WRIGHT

Bristol
1986

Published
under the Wright Imprint by IOP Publishing Limited, Techno House, Redcliffe Way, Bristol BS1 6NX

First edition, 1983
Second edition, 1986

British Library Cataloguing in Publication Data
Darke, P. G. G.
    Notes on canine internal medicine.—
    2nd ed.—(A veterinary practitioner handbook)
    1.   Dogs—Diseases
    I.   Title   II. Series
    636.7′0896   SF991

ISBN 0 7236 0887 3

(M) 636·708 a D

Typeset by
Severntype Repro Services Ltd,
Market Street, Wotton-under-Edge, Glos.

Printed in Great Britain by
Billing and Sons Ltd, Worcester

Preface to the Second Edition

The format of the First Edition of *Notes on Canine Internal Medicine* proved very successful, and is largely maintained for the Second Edition. However, in just three years, there has been sufficient progress in some fields, notably endocrinology, to justify some revision. Further attention has been paid to all references and the presentation of information within each chapter, with the continuing aim of presenting a ready-reference that is easily consulted, and packed with information. I hope that this book may stimulate clinicians to use thought rather than dogma, by presenting a diagnostic and therapeutic approach to problem cases in canine medicine. If this book helps to save a few lives or if it helps to protect some dogs against excessively prolonged investigation or inappropriate therapy, by providing fresh ideas, I shall be well pleased.

Since the preparation of this Edition, it is very sad to report our loss of a much-respected colleague and gentleman, Mr C. P. Mackenzie, to whom we owe a debt for developments in small animal medicine.

P. G. G. D.

Preface to the First Edition

During my early career in private veterinary practice, I was frequently frustrated by my lack of knowledge of the differential diagnosis, investigation and management of serious internal disorders in small animals. In the acceptance of medical cases referred to veterinary schools, I have recognized similar frustrations and limitations in my colleagues in the field. The thoracic and abdominal walls should not represent an iron curtain to clinicians with today's facilities and expertise.

This book is written to encourage a deeper understanding of the art of veterinary practice. I have tried to emphasize the most relevant clinical features of diseases of internal organs, and to present wherever possible, a simple step-by-step approach to the investigation of common clinical syndromes. However, a number of procedures suggested here may be beyond the facilities available to private practitioners, and arrival at this stage in an unresolved case may be an indication for referral to a centre with more facilities. *Confirmation* of many diagnoses requires biopsy, a feature of potentially increasing importance in the future. Many biopsy techniques are relatively simple and soon mastered.

Internal Medicine is here taken to include mainly the disorders of organs and systems of the pleural and peritoneal cavities. No attempt is made to describe the generalized infectious diseases, neurology, disorders of the head and neck, metabolic bone disease or reproductive disorders. A reasonable level of knowledge of canine medicine is assumed and detailed pathophysiology is avoided: this is already excellently covered by other authorities (*see* Bibliography *below*). I have tried to present facts in a plain fashion. Much is based on my opinion which may differ from that of other clinicians. I fully recognize that some subjects may be over-simplified and that many medical disorders fall into categories that are not so much black and white, but more a shade of grey. This is part of the challenge and stimulation of internal medicine for

Bibliography

Anderson N. V. (1980) *Veterinary Gastroenterology.* Philadelphia, Lea & Febiger.
Bovee K. C. (1984) *Canine Nephrology.* Harwall Publishing.
Catcott E. J. (1979) *Canine Medicine.* Santa Barbara, American Veterinary Publications.
Chandler E. A., Sutton J. B. and Thompson D. J. (1984) *Canine Medicine and Therapeutics,* 2nd ed. Oxford, Blackwell Scientific.
Ettinger S. J. (1983) *Textbook of Veterinary Internal Medicine: Diseases of the Dog and Cat.* Philadelphia, Saunders. 2nd ed.
Kirk R. W. (1980) *Current Veterinary Therapy: Small Animal Practice.* 7th ed. Philadelphia, Saunders.
Osborne C. A., Low D. G. and Finco D. R. (1972) *Canine and Feline Urology.* Philadelphia, Saunders.
Siegel E. T. (1977) *Endocrine Diseases of the Dog.* Philadelphia, Lea & Febiger.

me as a physician. I hope that this book may increase job satisfaction for colleagues. I welcome criticism and comments.

It is acknowledged that extensive case investigation and management is expensive, but it cannot be over-stressed that basic careful history taking and thorough, and if necessary, repeated clinical examination are fundamental procedures that may yield a diagnosis in a complicated or unresolved case.

I am very grateful to many colleagues for their comments on this text, especially Messrs A. G. Burnie, G. R. Dobbie, C. P. Mackenzie, J. W. Simpson, K. L. Thoday and Miss S. M. Crispin, all of whom contributed significantly. My wife, Carole, was very tolerant and helpful in typing and retyping most of the manuscript.

P. G. G. D.

Contents

Chapter 1
Airway Disorders   1
  General Management of Airway Disorders
  (including coughing)   7

Chapter 2
Pulmonary Disorders   10
  Management of Pulmonary Disorders   13

Chapter 3
Pleural and Mediastinal Disorders   16
  Treatment of Pleural and Mediastinal
  Disorders   19

Chapter 4
Thoracic Trauma   22

Chapter 5
**Differential Diagnosis of Respiratory
Disorders**   25
  A. Dyspnoea   26
  B. Coughing   27
  C. Noise   28

Chapter 6
Investigation of Respiratory Disorders   29

Chapter 7
**Further Investigation of Respiratory
Disorders**   33

Chapter 8
Cardiac Disorders   41

Chapter 9
Cardiac Failure   57

Chapter 10
**Differential Diagnosis of Episodic Weakness
or Collapse**   65
  Diagnosis Procedure for Collapse   67
  Differential Diagnosis of Cyanosis   68

Chapter 11
Cardiac Rhythm and Dysrhythmias   70
  Therapy for Dysrhythmias   74

Chapter 12
Investigation of Cardiac Disease   77

Chapter 13
Further Investigation of Cardiac Disease   83

Chapter 14
Management of Cardiac Failure   91

Chapter 15
Cardiac Arrest and Resuscitation   99

Chapter 16
Oesophageal Disorders   102

Chapter 17
Gastric Disorders   105

Chapter 18
Differential Diagnosis of Vomiting   110

Chapter 19
**Investigation of Persistent Vomiting/
Regurgitation**   116

Chapter 20
Acute Abdominal Disorders   121

Chapter 21
Disorders of the Small Intestine   125

Chapter 22
Disorders of the Large Intestine   131
    Differential Diagnosis of Acute
    Haemorrhagic Diarrhoea   133

Chapter 23
**Differential Diagnosis and Management of
Persistent Diarrhoea**   134

Chapter 24
Hepatic Disorders   144
    Diagnosis of Hepatic Disorders   149
    General Management of Hepatic Disease
    and Failure   152
    Differential Diagnosis of Hepatomegaly   153

Chapter 25
**Differential Diagnosis and Investigation of
Jaundice**   155

Chapter 26
Splenic Disorders   157

Chapter 27
Pancreatic Disorders   159

Chapter 28
Renal Disorders 163

Chapter 29
Lower Urinary Tract Disorders 170

Chapter 30
Prostatic Disorders 177
General Signs and Management of
Prostatic Disease 179

Chapter 31
Differential Diagnosis of Haematuria 182
Investigation of Haematuria 183

Chapter 32
**Differential Diagnosis of Urinary
Incontinence** 185
Investigation of Urinary Incontinence 186

Chapter 33
Differential Diagnosis of Tenesmus 189
Investigation of Tenesmus 190

Chapter 34
Disorders of the Peritoneal Cavity 192
Investigation of Abdominal Enlargement 194

Chapter 35
**Radiographic Findings in Abdominal
Disorders** 196

Chapter 36
Endocrine Disorders 203

Chapter 37
Disorders of the Female Genital Tract 225

Chapter 38
Differential Diagnosis of Polydipsia 229
Investigation of Polydipsia 230

Chapter 39
**Differential Diagnosis of Thinness and Weight
Loss** 233
Investigation of Thinness and Weight Loss 234

Chapter 40
Autoimmune Disorders 236

Chapter 41
**Differential Diagnosis of Recurrent or
Persistent Pyrexia**   241
 Investigation of Persistent or Recurrent
 Pyrexia   242

Chapter 42
Anaemia   245
 Investigation of Anaemia   249
 Approach to Unaccountable Haemorrhage
 or Prolonged Bleeding   252

Chapter 43
Acute Poisoning   257
 Approach to Suspected Poisoning   259

Index   263

Chapter 1

Airway Disorders

A. AIRWAY OBSTRUCTION (*See also* Lane, 1982)

1. Trauma to larynx or trachea
   (animal bites, choke chains, road accidents).
2. Brachycephalic airway obstruction
   —stenotic nares, elongated soft palate, narrow larynx,
   secondary laryngeal collapse (especially Pekes, Bulldogs).
3. Tracheal collapse
   (middle-aged obese small dogs, especially Yorkshire Terriers).
4. Tonsillar enlargement:
   a. Tonsillitis (usually secondary to other infections).
   b. Neoplasia.
5. Laryngeal disorders:
   a. Laryngeal paralysis
   ('roarers'—common in ageing large breeds of dog)—
   especially Irish setter, Afghan, Labrador retriever
   (idiopathic, traumatic, neoplastic, hypothyroidism).
   b. Laryngeal hyperplasia (or neoplasia—rare).
   c. Laryngeal oedema (stings, allergy, brachycephalic breeds).
6. Nodules of *Filaroides osleri*
   (young dogs—often infected by the dam).
7. Foreign bodies
   (especially pharynx or lower airway—sticks, ears of corn).
8. Space-occupying lesions:
   a. Within the airway
   (*rare,* other than salivary cysts or in tonsils).
   b. Pressing on the airway:
      i. Abscesses (especially pharyngeal).
      ii. Thyroid neoplasms.

1

      iii. Thymic lymphosarcoma.
      iv. Hyperplastic or neoplastic lymph nodes.
       v. Other thoracic neoplasms.
      vi. Gross cardiac enlargement.
9. Bronchospasm ('asthma'—*rare* but often incorrectly diagnosed).
10. Bronchitis
(when very productive, secretions may obstruct the airway).
11. Oesophageal obstruction or dilatation pressing on the airway.
12. Congenital malformations: tracheal hypoplasia
(Bulldog, Boxer).
13. Fluid obstruction:
    a. Vomitus or regurgitated material
       —especially with megaloesophagus or oral misdosing.
    b. Acute pulmonary oedema (usually cardiogenic).
    c. Pulmonary or tracheal haemorrhage.

Signs

    a. Dyspnoea with *noise,* exacerbated by excitement or exercise—
    usually:
      i. Inspiratory if above the thoracic inlet (sighing/snoring/
        stridor).
      ii. Expiratory if involving the lower airway
        (asthmatic 'wheeze' or honking sound).
     iii. Both inspiratory and expiratory if at the thoracic inlet
        (rattling or wheezing sound).
     iv. Abolished by opening the mouth if nasal.
    b. Coughing—if irritant to the airway.
    c. Dysphonia—if a laryngeal disorder (disturbance in the voice).
    d. Dysphagia—if the pharynx or oesophagus is involved.
    e. Bubbling sounds, air hunger (if pulmonary oedema).

Findings

    a. Cyanosis, if severe obstruction.
    b. Tonsillar and pharyngeal lesions may be visible on simple
       visual inspection of the mouth.
    c. The origin of noise may be located with a stethoscope.
    d. Traumatic lesions, collapsing trachea, tumours or masses may
       be palpated if in the neck region
    e. Subcutaneous emphysema may be found in trauma.
    f. Signs of cardiac failure (Chapter 9)?

Investigations (*See also* Chapter 7)

   a. Radiology of the airway:
      i. Plain films demonstrate few lesions:
          Trauma, peritracheal masses and oesophageal disorders may be readily identified.
          Cardiogenic pulmonary oedema is characteristic (Chapter 13).
          Tracheal collapse or hypoplasia
          (but collapse is poorly demonstrated on plain films).
          Nodules of *Filaroides osleri* are not usually visible.
      ii. Fluoroscopy is essential for diagnosis of some disorders, especially tracheal collapse.
      iii. Bronchography (Webbon & Clark), 1977.
   b. Laryngoscopy and bronchoscopy—p. 37:
      i. Very valuable in the diagnosis of some airway disorders: tonsillar lesions, laryngeal disorders, Filaroides, foreign bodies, intra-tracheal neoplasms.
      ii. May help in the diagnosis of chronic bronchitis, broncho-spasm, congenital deformities and tracheal collapse.
   c. Transtracheal washing (under local or general anaesthetic) for: cytology (leucocytes, eosinophils neoplastic cells), micro-biology, Filaroides larvae (Creighton and Wilkins, 1974).

Management (*See* General Aspects and Management of Coughing p. 7 and Lane, 1982)

   a. Acute and severe airway obstruction must be regarded as a *respiratory emergency:*
      i. The airway *must be cleared:*
          Clear the mouth/tongue/throat (suction if necessary).
          Lower the head.
          Intubate if unconscious.
          ? Anaesthetize (with care) and intubate if conscious.
          Do not sedate but i.v. atropine may be advised.
          ? Tracheotomy.
          Use a wide bore (e.g. 14 gauge) needle in emergency.
          Connect to oxygen supply?
      ii. Apply artificial respiration if respiratory arrest:
          blow down the endotracheal tube if necessary, or
          use an anaesthetic bag or ventilator (5–20 per min).
      iii. Consider the use of oxygen (25–40 per cent is ideal)
          But:
          Humidification of oxygen is desirable.

Usually not well tolerated by a distressed dog
Excessive oxygen may depress the ventilatory drive if
the dog is hypoxaemic.
? Bubble through alcohol if pulmonary oedema is present.

    iv. Supportive therapy:

Maintain warmth or cool (ice packs) if hyperthermic.
Maintain fluid intake—intravenously if necessary.
Antibiotics may be necessary to prevent secondary
pulmonary infection; corticosteroids may reduce
obstruction.

  b. *Bronchodilatation* if necessary:

    i. Xanthine derivatives (theophylline, aminophylline, etami-
phylline)—not very potent and must be administered
several times daily.

    ii. Atropine—also reduces secretions, though not advised in
cardiac failure.

    iii. β-adrenergic stimulants
terbutaline (Bricanyl; Astra) ⎫ but these are also
isoprenaline (Saventrine;   ⎬ cardiac stimulants
Pharmax)?   ⎭ (which may be
ephedrine   undesirable)

  c. *Coughing,* if it occurs, *see* p. 7.

Specific therapy

Surgical (Harvey, 1983)

  a. Traumatic lesions may require repair.
  b. Foreign bodies are removed via an endoscope or
surgically.
  c. Abscesses must be drained.
  d. Neoplasms are rarely simply removed.
  e. Obstructive Filaroides lesions can be removed via a
bronchoscope if necessary.
  f. Tracheal collapse has been treated by insertion of
prostheses and by plication of the dorsal membrane of
collapsed rings (Done, 1978).
  g. Arytenoid lateralization is indicated for laryngeal paralysis
(Lane, 1978).
  h. Brachycephalic breeds may benefit from surgery to the
nares, the soft palate and/or the larynx.

But surgical access and good healing are problematic for the
trachea.

Medical
  a. *Filaroides osleri, see* p. 6.
  b. Pulmonary oedema and cardiomegaly
     —diuresis is of prime importance—*see* Chapter 14.
  c. Brachycephalic airway obstruction—relief may be obtained with:
     i. Sedation.
     ii. Corticosteroids—betamethasone (Betsolan; Glaxo) (Diuretics may also help).
  d. Bronchospasm (asthma, allergic bronchitis):
     i. Bronchodilatation (p. 4).
     ii. Corticosteroids—parenterally, then orally for 3–5 days.

B. AIRWAY INFLAMMATION

Canine respiratory infections may be due to adenovirus, parainfluenza, distemper or herpes virus with *Bordetella bronchiseptica* as a primary or secondary pathogen. These generally cause tracheobronchitis, but laryngitis, pharyngitis and rhinitis occur in some cases. Failure to recover may lead to chronic bronchitis, bronchiectasis or bronchopneumonia, especially if secondary infection occurs.

1. Acute tracheobronchitis due to infection ('kennel cough').
2. Inflammation due to foreign bodies or irritants (smoke, dust, pollutants).
3. Chronic tracheobronchitis due to *Filaroides osleri:*
     Young dogs are most often affected.
     Direct infection occurs from the dam or other dogs.
4. Chronic bronchitis (or bronchiectasis)
     —may result from chronic infection, irritation or inflammation.
     Effects:
     a. Excess mucus production.
     b. Mucus stasis, loss of ciliary action.
     c. Narrowing of airways.
5. Laryngitis—may result from infection or persistent barking.
6. Inflammation may also be secondary to:
     a. Airway obstruction (tracheal collapse).
     b. Coughing—whatever the cause.
     c. Regurgitation or laryngeal dysfunction.

Signs
  a. Coughing:
     i. Often dry and paroxysmal, occasionally soft and persistent.

      ii. Noted especially: when animal awakes or is stimulated; with excitement or exercise.
- *b.* Dysphonia—if the larynx is involved.
- *c.* Oculonasal discharge ⎱ with some infections.
  Anorexia, depression ⎰
- *d.* 'Reverse sneeze' in rhinitis.

Findings

- *a.* Cough provoked by tracheal pinch?
- *b.* Pharyngitis/tonsillitis and pyrexia with some infections.
- *c.* Harsh rhonchi on auscultation? (Chapter 6).

Auscultation is often unrewarding, with non-specific findings.

Investigations

- *a.* Radiography (often unrewarding).
- *b.* Bronchoscopy and tracheoscopy (very valuable, Chapter 7).
- *c.* Faeces for Filaroides larvae (but larvae may not be present).
- *d.* Other tests (e.g. routine haematology) usually of little value.
- *e.* Tracheal or bronchial wash: for cytology, microbiology (Creighton and Wilkins, 1974).
- *f.* Bronchography (especially for bronchiectasis) (Webbon and Clarke, 1977).

Treatment

For general management of coughing *see* p. 7.
- *a.* Kennel cough, laryngitis and other tracheitis:
  - i. Often resolve without therapy.
  - ii. Symptomatic relief of coughing (q.v.) may help.
  - iii. Antibiotics penetrate the airway mucosa very poorly but they may be used to avoid or to relieve bronchopneumonia, especially if the dog is unwell.
  - iv. Vaccination (against some infectious agents) is available.
- *b. Filaroides osleri:*
  - i. Obstructive lesions can be removed surgically.
  - ii. Effective parasiticides include:
    - Levamisole (7·5 mg/kg orally for 3 weeks).
    - Albendazole (25 mg/kg orally for 5 days).
    - Fenbendazole (20 mg/kg orally for 3 weeks).
  - iii. In-contact dogs should be checked for infection.

     iv. Kennels should be thoroughly cleaned.
- c. Chronic bronchitis or bronchiectasis. No certain cure, but *see* general notes on coughing (p. 7); the following may help:
  - i. Expectorants or mucolytics.
  - ii. Vaporization/nebulization (Bemis and Appel, 1977).
  - iii. Antibiotics and corticosteroids—in relapses?
  - iv. Cough suppressants?—when the cough is distressing.
  - v. Bronchodilatation—if airway obstruction (p. 4).

N.B. *Client communication* is important (especially in *c*) as these are persistent or recurrent disorders with little certainty of a cure.

GENERAL MANAGEMENT OF AIRWAY DISORDERS

1. Environmental:
   - a. Minimize exercise—*rest* is important.
   - b. Avoid (i) irritant or dry atmosphere (smoke, dust, pollen, etc.); (ii) undue excitement.
   - c. Reduce obesity.
2. Ensure airway patency (*see* p. 3).

Coughing

Productive coughing is valuable and necessary to remove materials from the airway—especially with infections and bronchiectasis.
    Expectoration may be encouraged:
- a. Expectorants (eucalyptus, citrates, ammonium chloride).
- b. Mucolysis—bromhexine (Bisolvon; Boehringer).
- c. Use of nebulizers or bronchial washings?
- d. Use of steaming atmosphere (e.g. a shower room).
- e. Application of physiotherapy?

Unproductive coughing is usually undesirable:
- a. It may disseminate disease (infection, foreign body) into the lungs and to other animals.
- b. It is tiring and distressing (to animal and owner).
- c. It may cause secondary disease (e.g. emphysema, hypoxia, cor pulmonale, bronchiectasis, perineal rupture).

General therapeutic principles
- a. Discourage irritation:
  - i. *See* (1) *above.*
  - ii. Apply a shoulder harness rather than a collar to the dog.
  - iii. Use demulcents (honey, glycerol, menthol).
  - iv. Use corticosteroids in short courses.
  - v. Use antihistamines?

    b. Encourage bronchodilatation (*see* p. 4).
    c. Sedation and analgesia:
        i. Opiates (codeine, morphine, dextromethorphan).
        ii. Chloroform.
        iii. Antihistamines
        iv. Barbiturates.
    d. Antibacterial agents—penetrate the airway very poorly, but facilitated by bromhexine (Bisolvon; Boehringer).
    e. Treat cardiac failure (Ch. 14) or any specific disease (p. 6–7).

Therapeutic agents are often combined in proprietary cough medicines.

REFERENCES AND FURTHER READING

Bedford P. G. C. (1983) Displacement of the glosso-epiglottic mucosa in canine asphyxiate disease. *J. Small Anim. Pract.* **24,** 199.

Bemis D. A. and Appel M. J. G. (1977) Aerosol, parenteral and oral antibiotic treatment of *Bordetella bronchiseptica* infections in dogs. *J. Am. Vet. Med. Assoc.* **170,** 1082.

Bojrab M. J. and Nafe L. L. (1976) Tracheal reconstructive surgery. *J. Am. Anim. Hosp. Assoc.* **12,** 622.

Creighton S. R. and Wilkins R. J. (1974) Transtracheal aspiration biopsy: technique and cytologic evaluation. *J. Am. Anim. Hosp. Assoc.* **10,** 219.

Darke P. G. G. (1976) Use of levamisole in the treatment of parasitic tracheobronchitis in the dog. *Vet. Rec.* **99,** 293.

Dobbie G. R., Darke P. G. G. and Head K. W. (1986) Intrabronchial foreign bodies in dogs. *J. Small Anim. Pract.* **27,** 227.

Done S. H. (1978) Canine tracheal collapse—aetiology, pathology, diagnosis and treatment. In: Grunsell C. S. G. and Hill F. W. G. (ed.), *Veterinary Annual.* Bristol, Wright Scientechnica.

Ettinger S. J. and Ticer J. W. (1983) Diseases of the trachea. In: Ettinger S. J. (ed.), *Textbook of Veterinary Internal Medicine,* 2nd Ed. Philadelphia, Saunders.

Gaber C. E., Amis T. C. and LeCouteur R. A. (1985) Laryngeal paralysis in dogs: a review of 23 cases. *J. Am. Vet. Med. Assoc.* **186,** 377.

Harvey C. E. (1983) Review of results of airway obstruction surgery in the dog. *J. Small Anim. Pract.* **24,** 555.

Harvey C. E. and O'Brien J. A. (1972) Management of respiratory emergencies in small animals. *Vet. Clin. N. Am.* **2**(2), 243.

Lane J. G. (1978) Canine laryngeal surgery. In: Grunsell C. S. G. and Hill F. W. G. (ed.), *Veterinary Annual.* Bristol, Wright Scientechnica.

Lane J. G. (1982) *ENT and Oral Surgery of the Dog and Cat.* Bristol, Wright·PSG.

Lau R. E., Schwartz A. and Buergelt C. D. (1980) Tracheal resection and anastomosis in dogs. *J. Am. Vet. Med. Assoc.* **176,** 134.

O'Brien J. A. (1970) Bronchoscopy in the dog and cat. *J. Am. Vet. Med. Assoc.* **156,** 213.

Webbon P. M. and Clarke K. W. (1977) Bronchography in normal dogs. *J. Small Anim. Pract.* **18,** 327.

Wheeldon E. B., Pirie H. M., Fisher E. W. et al. (1974) Chronic bronchitis in the dog. *Vet. Rec.* **94,** 466.

Wheeldon E. B., Suter P. F. and Jenkin T. (1982) Neoplasia of the larynx of the dog. *J. Am. Vet. Med. Assoc.* **180**, 642.

Wright N. G., Thompson H., Cornwall H. J. et al. (1974) Canine respiratory virus infections. *J. Small Anim. Pract.* **15**, 27.

Wykes P. M. (1983) Canine laryngeal diseases. Part I Anatomy and disease syndromes. *Comp. Continuing Ed. Pract. Vet.* **8**, 8.

Chapter 2

Pulmonary Disorders

A. ALVEOLAR DISEASES

1. Haemorrhage:
   a. A common sequel to road accidents (Chapter 4).
   b. With coagulopathies (Chapter 42).
   c. From neoplasms (e.g. haemangiosarcoma).
2. Oedema—usually caused by:
     i. raised capillary pressure
    ii. increased capillary permeability.
   a. Common sequel to congestive cardiac failure (Chapter 9).
   b. Toxic (e.g. ANTU, paraquat poisoning, inhaled smoke).
   c. Drowning, heat stroke, electric shock.
   d. Shock (an uncommon cause in dogs).
   e. ? Allergic (uncommon).
   f. Secondary to other disorders
      (e.g. pneumonia or hypoproteinaemias).
   g. Neurogenic (e.g. CNS trauma or encephalitis) (uncommon).
   h. Intravenous fluid overload (uncommon in dogs).
3. Exudation—bronchopneumonia, usually secondary to:
   a. Airway infections
      (common agents: Pseudomonas, Pasteurellae, streptococci).
   b. Inhalation of irritants
      (e.g. careless dosing; regurgitation—megaloesophagus).
   c. Lung lobe collapse/consolidation. (Neoplasia/foreign body/
      exudate obstructing a bronchus).
4. Neoplasia (primary carcinoma in ageing dogs) may cause:
   a. Bronchial obstruction.
   b. Lung lobe collapse.

      c. Infection/emphysema.
      d. Pleural effusion (Chapter 3).
     May metastasize within the lungs.
     May cause HPOA (Marie's disease) (p.19).
  5. Emphysema:
      a. Occurs quite commonly with bronchitis.
      b. Occasionally occurs with other bronchial obstructions.
      c. Idiopathic (especially West Highland White Terrier?).
  6. Granulomatous infections (not common):
     fungi, tuberculosis, toxoplasmosis.
  7. Allergic (eosinophilic) pneumonia—may be seasonal /parasitic?

Signs

      a. Dyspnoea (shallow tachypnoea) according to severity.
      b. Coughing—often soft, moist and productive if (1), (2) or (3).
      c. Nasal discharge
         —if very productive and in brachycephalic breeds.
      d. Exercise intolerance.
      e. Debility—fatigue, weight loss, poor appetite.
      f. Lameness/swelling of limbs—if HPOA (p.19).
      g. (Other haemorrhages with coagulopathies.)

Findings

      a. Cyanosis if severe.
      b. (Pale mucous membranes with shock or haemorrhage.)
      c. Auscultation (*see* Chapter 6):
         i. Pulmonary râles—may be localized.
        ii. Vesicular sounds may or may not be present.
       iii. Rhonchi may be present if airways are involved.
       iv. Respiratory sounds may be displaced ⎫
           heart sounds may be muffled   ⎬ by masses.
      d. Chronic disease may cause HPOA (p.19).

Investigations

      a. Radiography is of prime importance (Chapter 7).
      b. For cardiac failure: *see* Chapters 12 and 13.
      c. Haematology:
         i. Leucocytosis in bronchopneumonia.
        ii. Anaemia (with regeneration) in haemorrhagic disorders.
       iii. ? Polycythaemia in chronic disorders.
       iv. Eosinophilia in allergic pneumonia.

B. PULMONARY INTERSTITIAL DISEASES

1. Viral pneumonia (distemper, adenovirus).
2. Neoplasia—common site for *metastases* from:
   - *a.* Mammary neoplasms.
   - *b.* Osteosarcomas.
   - *c.* Melanomas (mouth, digits).
   - *d.* Carcinomas.
   - *e.* Haemangiosarcomas.
   - *f.* Occasionally the site for diffuse lymphosarcoma.
3. Parasitic infections:
   - *a.* Migrating ascarid larvae.
   - *b.* *Angiostrongylus vasorum* (especially Greyhounds).
   - *c.* (*Dirofilaria imitis*—imported dogs.)
4. Paraquat poisoning—causes fibrosis and other severe changes (fatal, after several days' progressive dyspnoea).
5. Pulmonary oedema (especially congestive cardiac failure).

Signs

- *a.* Dyspnoea (tachypnoea) when the lesion is widespread.
- *b.* (Rarely coughing—unproductive if it occurs.)
- *c.* Weight loss in chronic disorders (neoplasia, infections).
- *d.* Vomiting and anorexia occur early in paraquat poisoning.

Findings

Often minimal—it may be difficult to make a specific diagnosis:
- *a.* Cyanosis occurs if the disease is severe.
- *b.* Oral ulceration occurs in paraquat poisoning.

Investigations

- *a.* Radiography is of prime importance (Chapter 7). *But* interstitial pneumonia and paraquat poisoning may produce few changes.
- *b.* Lung biopsy is indicated for pathological diagnosis (Chapter 7).

C. MISCELLANEOUS PULMONARY DISEASES

Numerous other disorders are occasionally found:
1. Lung lobe torsion (producing dyspnoea and pleural effusion).
2. Lung lobe rupture—especially bullae (causes acute pneumothorax).

3. Lung lobe collapse (atelectasis) following bronchial obstruction or lung compression by pleural or pulmonary masses or fluid.
4. Granulomatous diseases—may cause abscessation:
   a. Fungal or tubercular infections.
   b. Toxoplasmosis or Angiostrongylus.
   c. Foreign bodies (grass awns).
5. Pulmonary vascular disorders:
   a. Embolism and pulmonary thrombosis—may be associated with amyloidosis or parasitic infections (Angiostrongylus or Dirofilaria) (difficult to diagnose *in vivo*).
   b. Congenital:
      i. Pulmonary arteriovenous shunts—may cause cyanosis.
      ii. Pulmonary artery stenosis.

Signs and investigations

Similar to those in interstitial disease.
Prognosis is generally poor.

MANAGEMENT OF PULMONARY DISORDERS

General therapy—of prime importance:
   a. Keep the airway patent.
   b. Encourage complete rest and maintain warmth.
   c. Encourage productive coughing if accumulated materials are not otherwise readily removed (e.g. bronchopneumonia) (p. 7).
   d. Encourage drainage from lungs:
      i. By posture (lying the dog with the forequarters lowered).
      ii. With physiotherapy?
Ensure adequate fluid intake, especially if animal is dyspnoeic— because dyspnoea may:
      i. Cause excessive fluid loss.
      ii. Discourage the dog from drinking.
Oxygen therapy may be necessary in emergency (Chapter 1).
N.B. repeated radiographs may be a valuable guide to progress.

Specific therapy
   a. Surgical resection may be indicated for:
      i. Lung lobe torsion.
      ii. Primary neoplasm—but usually too extensive and malignant.
      iii. Abscesses or granulomas?
      iv. Ruptured bullae.

Requires thoracotomy and postive-pressure ventilation.

  b. Parasitic infections—anthelmintics may be valuable:
    i. Levamisole (7·5 mg/kg orally, daily for 3 weeks).
    ii. Albendazole (25 mg/kg orally for 5 days).
    iii. Fenbendazole (20 mg/kg orally for 3 weeks).
  c. Oedema—for therapy for cardiac failure (*see* Chapter 14):
    i. Diuresis (frusemide or thiazides) is very valuable.
    ii. Xanthine derivatives (aminophylline, etamiphylline) may help— but not very potent.
  d. Bronchopneumonia (also interstitial pneumonia or abscess) requires antibiotic therapy at high levels at least twice daily for at least 2 weeks—a slow response suggests:
    i. Bronchial obstruction (neoplasm, foreign body).
    ii. Inappropriate antibacterial treatment.
    iii. Other systemic disease (cardiac or renal failure).
    iv. Secondary disease—abscessation or pyothorax.
    Bromhexine (Bisolvon; Boehringer) aids clearance of exudates.
  e. Haemorrhage is usually rapidly self-resolving with care and nursing but:
    i. If it is recurrent, reconsider the cause (coagulopathy, trauma or neoplasia?)
    ii. Antibiotic therapy is advisable to prevent secondary infection.
  f. Metastatic neoplasia and paraquat poisoning carry a hopeless prognosis and no successful treatment is currently available.
  g. Allergic pneumonia: alternate-day prednisolone therapy may be required when the disease is severe.

REFERENCES AND FURTHER READING

Berzon J. L., Rendano V. T. and Hoffer R. E. (1979) Recurrent pneumothorax secondary to ruptured pulmonary blebs: a case report. *J. Am. Anim. Hosp. Assoc.* **15,** 707.
Brodey R. S. (1971) Hypertrophic osteoarthropathy in the dog: a clinicopathologic survey of 60 cases *J. Am. Vet. Med. Assoc.* **159,** 1242.
Brodey R. S. (1979) Aspects of hypertrophic osteoarthropathy. In: Grunsell C. S. G. and Hill F. W. G. (ed.), *Veterinary Annual.* Bristol, Wright Scientechnica.
Brodey R. S. and Craig P. H. (1965) Primary pulmonary neoplasms in the dog: a review of 29 cases. *J. Am. Vet. Med. Assoc.* **147,** 1628.
Lord P. F. (1975) Neurogenic pulmonary edema in the dog. *J. Am. Anim. Hosp. Assoc.* **11,** 778.
Lord P. F. (1976) Alveolar lung diseases in small animals and their radiographic diagnosis. *J. Small Anim. Pract.* **17,** 283.
Lord P. F., Greiner T. P., Greene R. W. et al. (1973) Lung lobe torsion in the dog. *J. Am. Anim. Hosp. Assoc.* **9,** 473.

Lynch V. (1977) *Angiostrongylus vasorum* in the dog. *Vet. Rec.* **101,** 41.

McKiernon B. C. (1983). Lower respiratory tract diseases. In: Ettinger S. J. (ed.), *Textbook of Veterinary Internal Medicine,* 2nd Ed. Philadelphia, Saunders.

Orsher A. N. R. and Kolata R. J. (1982) Acute respiratory distress syndrome: case report and literature review. *J. Am. Anim. Hosp. Assoc.* **18,** 41.

Reif J. S. (1969) Solitary pulmonary lesions in small animals. *J. Am. Vet. Med. Assoc.* **155,** 717.

Chapter 3

Pleural and Mediastinal Disorders

A. EFFUSIONS

Small quantities of serous fluids perfuse body cavities naturally, and accumulation represents an upset in the balance between diffusion and absorption, or the active secretion or release of materials. Pleural effusions are *common*. Careful investigation is important.

1. Blood (haemothorax) (Chapter 42):
   a. Traumatic (Chapter 4).
   b. From neoplasms (e.g. haemangiosarcoma).
   c. Coagulopathies (warfarin, hepatic failure, platelet disorders).
   d. Others: pulmonary thrombosis, lung lobe torsion.
2. Pus (mediastinitis, exudative pleurisy).
   The cause is often uncertain—it includes:
   a. Penetration (bite wounds, traumatic, foreign body)—of the thorax/oesophagus/airway.
   b. Pleural foreign body (grass seed, stick, gunshot).
   c. Spread from lungs or mediastinum—typical agents: Nocardia, streptococci, staphylococci, (TB), *Bacteroides* spp.
   d. Surgery.
3. Chyle:
   a. Traumatic rupture of lymphatics.
   b. Neoplastic obstruction or erosion of the thoracic duct.
   c. Idiopathic or pseudochylous—in many cases.
4. Modified transudate (Chapter 7)
   (due to raised capillary hydrostatic pressure):
   a. Congestive or right-sided cardiac failure.
   b. Neoplastic obstruction of venous return (e.g. heart base tumour).

16

    c. Ruptured diaphragm.

    d. Lung lobe torsion.

    e. Thoracic adhesions.

5. True transudate (Chapter 7) (associated with hypoproteinaemias):

    a. Renal loss (glomerulonephritis).

    b. Alimentary loss (e.g. lymphangiectasia).

    c. Malabsorption or hepatic failure.

    May also arise from increased capillary permeability.

6. Other effusions:

    a. Neoplastic (e.g. carcinomatosis or mesothelioma).

    b. Biliary (liver through ruptured diaphragm).

7. Air (pneumothorax):

    a. Traumatic.

    b. Spontaneous, especially from blebs or bullae in lungs.

    c. Ruptured airway or oesophagus (foreign body, tumour).

    Pneumomediastinum is also an occasional sequel to trauma or severe dyspnoea.

Effusions are usually bilateral in dogs.

Clinical signs are usually noted only when large quantities have accumulated.

Signs

    a. Dyspnoea (tachypnoea), especially when the animal is stressed.

    b. Abnormal posture: standing or sternal recumbency, with elbows abducted.

    c. Weight loss (especially if chronic), depression, anorexia.

    d. Unwillingness to exercise.

    e. (Occasionally—coughing.)

    f. Abdominal enlargement—if ascites are also present.

Findings

    a. Pallor of mucous membranes and a weak pulse—(if acute haemorrhage).

    b. Cyanosis, especially when the animal is handled or stressed.

    c. Percussion:

       i. If pneumothorax: increased resonance

      ii. If fluid effusion: increased dorsal resonance with ventral dullness.

    d. Auscultation:

       i. Muffling of cardiac sounds.

      ii. Evidence of cardiac failure (Chapter 12)?

     iii. Dorsal displacement of respiratory sounds.

    e. Subcutaneous oedema (hypoproteinaemia)?
N.B. Repeated haemorrhage may occur in the presence of
neoplasia.

Investigations

N.B. A dyspnoeic animal must be handled with *care.*

    a. Radiography confirms the diagnosis:
        i. An erect or standing lateral film is helpful.
        ii. The dorsoventral position may be safer than
           ventrodorsal.
        iii. Check for neoplasms/cardiac enlargement.
    b. *Paracentesis* following antisepsis and local analgesia
       (Chapter 7).
    c. Laboratory tests: routine haematology, total and differential
       proteins, and urinalysis may be helpful (Chapter 7).
    d. Thoracotomy may be necessary to confirm or identify a
       lesion.
    e. Examine effusive fluid in detail (Chapter 7).

B. SPACE-OCCUPYING LESIONS

1. Structures herniated through a ruptured diaphragm
   (or through a congenital pericardiodiaphragmatic hernia).
2. Gross cardiomegaly.
3. Gross oesophageal dilatation (megaloesophagus).
4. Lymphomegaly—inflammatory, neoplastic, granulomatous.
5. Aortic body ('heart base') tumour.
6. Thymic lymphosarcoma.
7. (Thymoma—may be associated with myasthenia gravis.)
8. Other mediastinal neoplasms and abscesses.

Signs (only if the lesion is sufficiently large)

    a. Dyspnoea.
    b. Respiratory noise (if the airway is obstructed).
    c. Oedema of neck, head and forelimbs (if venous return is
       affected).
    d. Regurgitation (if pressure on the oesophagus or if
       megaloesophagus).

Findings (very variable)

    a. An area of dullness may be detected by percussion (mass/fluid).

    b. Heart sounds may be muffled or displaced mass/fluid.

    c. Respiratory sounds may be muffled or displaced.

    d. Occasionally, the distal limbs are painful and swollen—
if exostoses of hypertrophic pulmonary osteoarthropathy
(HPOA or Marie's disease) are present.

    e. Pleural effusion.

Investigations

    a. Radiography is essential—barium may outline the position of
the oesophagus in relation to a suspected lesion

    b. Paracentesis is required if effusion is present (Chapter 7).

    c. Thoracotomy or needle biopsy (using local anaesthesia and a
Tru-Cut needle (Travenol) may be needed to identify a
lesion.

TREATMENT OF PLEURAL AND MEDIASTINAL DISORDERS

General aspects

    a. Other than thymoma, most pleural or mediastinal masses are
malignant and inoperable.

    b. The prognosis for many disorders causing pleural effusions is
poor. However, repeated drainage may be necessary for
diagnosis and symptomatic treatment (Chapter 7).

    c. *Rest* and careful handling are essential for any dog with
dyspnoea.

Specific therapy

    a. Pyothorax—repeated drainage or the use of an indwelling
catheter or chest drain is essential (*see* p. 40), together with:

        i. Intensive antibacterial therapy:

            Initially with broad-spectrum agents (e.g. amoxycillin
or ampicillin) then according to bacterial sensitivity
—given parenterally, frequently and over several
weeks,
—given locally (soluble preparations) into the
thorax.
Clindamycin may be most effective in nocardiosis.
Metronidazole (20 mg/kg/day) may also be needed
for anaerobes.

        ii. Thoracic lavage (is probably of doubtful value).

    iii. Thoracotomy to break down adhesions if 'pocketing' of pus?—or fibrinolytic agents (e.g. Streptokinase (Varidase; Lederle)) intrapleurally *but* their use is painful and distressing.

    iv. Potassium iodide B.P. 5 mg/kg body weight orally daily for 2–3 weeks for nocardiosis.

Early diagnosis and treatment probably aid success.

  b. Pleural effusion of cardiac failure—*see* Chapter 14.

  c. Pneumothorax: rapid resolution is common without treatment. *But,* if a leak is persistent, a drainage tube and an underwater seal may be helpful, or repeated aspiration may be necessary while a lesion is healing. A Heimlich valve or water trap may help.

  d. Haemothorax—drainage is required if the dog has dyspnoea, *but* if blood is not removed, materials may be re-employed by the body for erythropoiesis or re-administered intravenously ('autotransfusion').

  e. Chylothorax—repeated drainage may be required and the prognosis guarded, but:

    i. The disorder may resolve spontaneously.

    ii. Thoracotomy to tie off a lesion or the thoracic duct is possible, but very difficult.

    iii. A diet low in fats will help to minimize this effusion.

  f. Neoplastic effusions are rarely curable.

  g. Ruptured diaphragm can usually be repaired by an abdominal surgical approach, with careful anaesthesia to support respirations (Garson et al., 1980).

REFERENCES AND FURTHER READING

Ackerman N., Grain E. and Castleman W. (1982) Canine nocardiosis. *J. Am. Anim. Hosp. Assoc.* **18,** 147.

Aronsohn M. G., Schunk K. L., Carpenter J. L. and King N. W. (1984) Clinical and pathologic features of thymoma in 15 dogs. *J. Am. Vet. Med. Assoc.* **184,** 1355.

Bellah J. R., Stiff M. E. and Russell R. G. (1983) Thymoma in the dog: two case reports and review of 20 additional cases *J. Am. Vet. Med. Assoc.* **183,** 306.

Berg J. (1982) Chylothorax in dogs and cats. *Compend. Continuing Ed. Pract. Vet.* **4,** 986.

Berzon J. L., Rendano V. T. and Hoffer R. E. (1979) Recurrent pneumothorax secondary to ruptured pulmonary blebs: a case report. *J. Am. Anim. Hosp. Assoc.* **15,** 707.

Birchard S. J., Cantwell H. D. and Bright R. M. (1982) Lymphangiography and ligation of the canine thoracic duct. A study in normal dogs and three dogs with chylothorax. *J. Am. Anim. Hosp. Assoc.* **18,** 769.

Campbell B. and Scott D. W. (1975) Successful management of nocardial empyema in a dog and cat. *J. Am. Anim. Hosp. Assoc.* **11,** 769.

Creighton S. R. and Wilkins R. J. (1980) Pleural effusions. In: Kirk R. W. (ed.), *Current Veterinary Therapy VII.* Philadelphia, Saunders.

Garson H. L., Dodman N. H. and Barker G. J. (1980) Diaphragmatic hernia. Analysis of fifty-six cases in dogs and cats. *J. Small Anim. Pract.* **21,** 469.

Jones B. R., Bath M. L. and Wood A. K. W. (1974) Spontaneous pneumomediastinum in the racing greyhound. *J. Small Anim. Pract.* **15,** 27.

Quick C. B. (1980) Chylothorax: a review *J. Am. Anim. Hosp. Assoc. 16,* 23.

Robertson S. A., Stoddart M. E., Evans R. J., Gaskell C. J. and Gibbs C. (1983) Thoracic empyema in the dog; a report of twenty-two cases. *J. Small Anim. Pract.* **24,** 103.

Suter P. F. and Zinkl J. G. (1983) Mediastinal, pleural, extrapleural and miscellaneous thoracic diseases. In: Ettinger S. J. (ed.) *Textbook of Veterinary Internal Medicine,* 2nd Ed. Philadelphia, Saunders.

Chapter 4

Thoracic Trauma

Commonly results from road accidents.
Thoracic injury should always be considered in cases with severe trauma or forelimb fractures.

Disorders

  a. Intrapulmonary haemorrhage
      —very common, but often overlooked.
  b. Pneumothorax (from damage to airway, alveoli or the thoracic wall):
       i. Closed—self-limiting.
      ii. Open (chest wall penetration).
     iii. Tension (leaking from lungs with every respiration).
  c. Haemothorax.
  d. Thoracic wall injury—may be loss of firm structures (flail chest).
  e. Ruptured diaphragm (onset of signs may be delayed).
  f. Fractured ribs (painful, but may be overlooked).
  g. Other effusions—chyle (bile) (onset of signs may be delayed).
  h. Airway obstruction (haemorrhage, tracheal trauma).
  i. Cardiac trauma (myocardial contusion, haemopericardium).

General signs

  a. Dyspnoea
      —exaggerated attempts to breathe if there is airway obstruction.
  b. Respiratory noise—if airway obstruction.

  c. Often associated shock:
   i. Pale mucous membranes.
   ii. Depression.
  d. Pain/bruising/fractured ribs/pneumothorax.
  e. Coughing (pulmonary haemorrhage or airway trauma).
  N.B. Skull and brain trauma can cause respiratory *depression*.

Findings

  a. Thoracic wall wounds.
  b. Increased *or* decreased resonance with percussion
     (ruptured diaphragm/haemothorax/pneumothorax).
  c. Muffled/displaced heart and respiratory sounds.
  d. Cyanosis, especially if pulmonary expansion is restricted.
  e. Subcutaneous emphysema (occasionally).
  f. Empty abdomen and alimentary sounds in the thorax
     (ruptured diaphragm).
  g. Dysrhythmias (myocardial trauma or shock).

Investigations

Radiology (Chapter 7) with *care* in handling. Radiographs must be
carefully examined for all features listed under 'Disorders' above.

Treatment

  a. *Immediate:*
   i. Ensure a patent airway (Chapter 1):
        Draw the tongue forward, clear the mouth.
        Suction/posture/intubation required?
   ii. Administer oxygen—or anaesthetize and ventilate.
   iii. Control any severe haemorrhage.
   iv. Ensure that the thoracic wall is intact.
   v. Administer intravenous fluids for shock
        (colloids rather than saline)
        (with *care* if pulmonary or pericardial haemorrhage).
   vi. Monitor closely.
  b. *Less urgent:*
   i. Drain haemothorax or pneumothorax
        but these may be self-resolving if not severe.
   ii. Surgery to repair ruptured diaphragm or thoracic wall.
   iii. Give support:
        Rest and warmth.
          Analgesia (*care* with opiates, as these depress
            respirations).
          Antibiotics (?) to prevent bronchopneumonia.

REFERENCES AND FURTHER READING

Garson H. L., Dodman N. H. and Baker G. J. (1980) Diaphragmatic hernia. Analysis of fifty-six cases in dogs and cats. *J. Small. Anim. Pract.* **21**, 469.

Hall L. W. (1964) The accident case V. The diagnosis of thoracic injuries. *J. Small Anim. Pract.* **5**, 35.

Harvey C. E. and O'Brien J. A. (1972) Management of respiratory emergencies in small animals. *Vet. Clin. N. Am.* **2**, 243.

Krahwinkel D. J. (1980) Thoracic trauma. In: Kirk R. W. (ed.), *Current Veterinary Therapy VII.* Philadelphia, Saunders.

Roenigk W. J. (1971) Injuries to the thorax. *J. Am. Anim. Hosp. Assoc.* **7**, 266.

Walker R. G. (1959) Traumatic pneumothorax in small animals. *Vet. Rec.* **71**, 859.

Chapter 5

Differential Diagnosis of Respiratory Disorders

Major signs of respiratory disease include:

Dyspnoea (difficulty in breathing)

a. Tachypnoea (rapid)—many pulmonary or pleural disorders—may be shallow or heaving—with marked respiratory effort.
b. Hyperpnoea (increased depth) (especially with obstructions).
c. Orthopnoea (sternal recumbency, elbows abducted).

Dyspnoea usually represents *severe* disease, because:

i. Changes in the character of respirations are not obvious to a client until disease is severe or widespread.
ii. Considerable respiratory reserve capacity has been exhausted.
iii. Animals compensate for respiratory disease by becoming less active.

Coughing

Produced by airway irritation (between the pharynx and bronchioles) (rarely, by pleurisy).

It is very readily provoked by only *mild* disease.

Coughing may be described as:

a. Dry and paroxysmal (e.g. Filaroides, smoke irritation).
b. Soft and productive (e.g. bronchopneumonia, haemorrhage).
c. Honking and wheezing (with noise—e.g. tracheal collapse).

But many disorders produce similar or varying coughs.

Respiratory noise

Produced by airway obstructions:

a. Inspiratory noise—cranial to the thoracic inlet.
b. Expiratory noise—caudal to the thoracic inlet.
—may be stridor, wheeze, whistle, gurgle, sighing.

Dysphonia

Changes in voice accompany laryngeal disorders.

A. DIFFERENTIAL DIAGNOSIS OF DYSPNOEA

1. Airway obstruction

Usually also causing noise. (There may also be cyanosis and coughing):
- a. Foreign body, neoplasm, trauma.
- b. Laryngeal paralysis/collapse/oedema ('roarer').
- c. Soft palate overlength/oedema (*see* Lane, 1982).
- d. Tracheal collapse.
- e. Filaroides infection.
- f. Bronchiectasis.
- g. Masses pressing on the airway:
  - i. Tumours (thyroid/lymphoid/heart base/thymic).
  - ii. Abscesses.
  - iii. Gross cardiomegaly.
- h. Asthma/bronchospasm (uncommon).
- i. Nasal disorders (*see* Lane, 1982).

2. Loss of thoracic capacity

Usually tachypnoea/dyspnoea, especially when the dog is stressed (occasionally also cyanosis):
- a. Effusions:
  - i. Haemorrhage/chyle/pus.
  - ii. True or modified transudates.
  - iii. Air.
  - iv. Neoplastic.
  - v. (Bile)
- b. Ruptured diaphragm
  (or congenital pericardiodiaphragmatic hernia).
- c. Mediastinal/pleural tumours.
- d. Intra-abdominal masses/ascites/gastric dilatation/pregnancy pressing on the diaphragm.
- e. Gross cardiomegaly.

3. Loss of pulmonary capacity for gaseous exchange

Usually shallow tachypnoea. (Cyanosis occurs if disease is severe.):
- a. Pulmonary oedema (especially in cardiac failure).
- b. Metastatic neoplasia (or primary neoplasia).
- c. Intrapulmonary haemorrhage.
- d. Bronchopneumonia.
- e. Paraquat poisoning.
- f. (Pulmonary thrombosis.)
- g. Pulmonary emphysema.

4. Physiological/metabolic

   a. Physiological (often *open-mouthed* panting):
- i. Hyperthermia/heat stroke.
- ii. Obesity.
- iii. Excitement/fright/nervousness.
- iv. Parturition/false pregnancy.

   b. Secondary:
- i. Pain, fever.
- ii. Shock, acidosis.
- iii. Anaemia/hypoxia.
- iv. Eclampsia.
- v. CNS disorders (encephalitis/trauma).
- vi. Endocrine disturbances.
   (phaeochromocytoma/hyperthyroidism).

Dyspnoeas are best investigated by radiology (Chapter 7).

B. DIFFERENTIAL DIAGNOSIS OF COUGHING

1. Acute

   a. Kennel cough (tracheobronchitis).
   b. Airway irritation (smoke/dust/chemicals).
   c. Airway trauma
   d. Airway foreign body.
   e. Pulmonary haemorrhage.
   f. Inhalation pneumonia
   g. Allergic (eosinophilic) pneumonia.

2. Persistent or recurrent

   a. Chronic bronchitis/bronchiectasis.
   b. Pulmonary congestion/oedema (left-sided cardiac failure).
   c. Filaroides infection.
   d. Tracheal collapse.
   e. Foreign body.
   f. Bronchopneumonia.
   g. Pulmonary neoplasia.
   h. Pressure on the airway.
   i. Brachycephalic airway obstruction.
   j. Allergic (eosinophilic) pneumonia.
   k. Recurrent inhalation (megaloesophagus/laryngeal/pharyngeal disorders).
   l. (Pleurisy.)
   m. (Tuberculosis.)

Chronic coughing is best investigated by bronchoscopy
(*See* p.37).

C. DIFFERENTIAL DIAGNOSIS OF
RESPIRATORY NOISE

1. **Inspiratory noise** (*see* Lane, 1982)
    a. Nose:
        i. Stenotic nares.
        ii. Neoplasms.
        iii. Trauma.
        iv. Foreign body.
        v. Natural 'snore'.
        vi. 'Reverse sneeze'.
    b. Pharynx.
        i. Soft palate elongation/oedema.
        ii. Tonsil hyperplasia/neoplasia.
        iii. Trauma (stick) injuries.
        iv. Brachycephalic airway obstruction.
    c. Larynx.
        i. Foreign body.
        ii. Paralysis ('roarer').
        iii. Trauma (dog bites).
        iv. Everted lateral ventricles.
        v. (Tumour/hyperplasia.)
    d. Trachea:
        i. Tracheal collapse.
        ii. Trauma.
        iii. Foreign body.
        iv. Tumours—compressing airway (thyroid/lymphoid)
            or within the airways (rare).
        v. Abscess—compressing airway.

2. **Expiratory noise**
    a. Tracheal collapse:
    b. Foreign body.
    c. Filaroides nodules.
    d. Masses (lymphoid/thymic/heart base).
    e. Enlarged heart.
    f. Bronchospasm/asthma.

REFERENCE AND FURTHER READING

Lane J. G. (1982) *ENT and Oral Surgery of the Dog and Cat.* Bristol, Wright PSG.

Chapter 6

Investigation of Respiratory Disorders

Respiratory disorders often require careful investigation. Instant 'spot' diagnosis and treatment are unlikely to yield fruitful results.

A. HISTORY

1. *Age:*
    a. Young—congenital disorder? infection?
    b. Older—neoplasia/bronchitis/cardiac failure?
2. Breed—e.g.:
    a. Boxer—neoplasia?
    b. Brachycephalics—airway obstruction?
    c. Yorkshire Terrier and toy breeds—tracheal collapse?
    d. West Highland White Terrier—pulmonary emphysema?
    e. Irish Setter—regurgitation and inhalation?
3. Vaccination status; any other dogs affected?
4. Respiratory signs:
    a. Cough, dyspnoea, respiratory noise?
    b. Previous episodes of dyspnoea, coughing or collapse?
    c. Nature, frequency and time of any coughing.
    d. Dysphonia (change in voice)?
       (Information is not usually volunteered by a client)?
5. Signs of upper respiratory tract infection
   (Oculonasal discharge, sneeze)?
6. Rate of onset and development:
    a. Slow and gradual
       (Neoplasia, chronic bronchitis, some pleural effusions.)

29

    b. Sudden
    (Trauma, foreign bodies, respiratory infections.)
    N.B. Dyspnoea may *appear* to be sudden, even if slow in
onset.
7. Environment:
    a. Urban—infection, irritants?
    b. Rural—foreign body, poison?
8. Possibility of:
    a. Trauma or fights (past or recent).
    b. Access to poisons (paraquat or warfarin).
    c. Heart disease.
    d. Contact with respiratory infections.
    (Recent kennelling/other dogs affected?).
    e. Previous removal of neoplasms.
    f. Dusty or smoky atmosphere.
9. General physical details:
    a. Weight loss, anorexia, lethargy (neoplasia, cardiac, effusion?)
    b. Previous history of illness (infections, neoplasia?)
    c. Regurgitation (oesophageal disease?).
    d. Exercise tolerance.

B. OBSERVATIONS

1. Physical condition: generalized or localized illness?
2. Rate and character of respiration:
   Depth/effort/rhythm (normal respiratory rate 10–30/min).
3. Shape and symmetry of nose/neck/chest.
4. Frequency and nature of coughing:
    a. After swallowing? (pharyngeal/laryngeal, oesophageal).
    b. Wheezy? (esp. at exercise—obstruction).
    c. Dry, with retch? (esp. nights and mornings—cardiac/
    bronchitis).
    d. Haemoptysis? (trauma/neoplasia/FB/coagulopathy/
    thrombosis.
5. Presence of respiratory noise
   (and whether inspiratory or expiratory).
6. Stance: does it indicate true dyspnoea?:
    a. Air hunger? (standing with neck extended, lips drawn).
    b. 'Barrel chest'? (in severe dyspnoea).
    c. Orthopnoea? (sternal recumbency, elbows abducted).
7. Other features:
    a. Lameness (due to HPOA, p. 19)?
    b. Horner's syndrome? if a cervical or thoracic lesion.

C. INSPECTION

1. Mucous membranes:
   a. Cyanosis (= hypoxia) (Chapter 10).
      i. Airway obstruction.
      ii. Severe pulmonary disorders.
      iii. Lack of thoracic capacity.
      iv. Cardiac right-to-left shunt.
   b. Pallor (haemorrhage or cardiac failure).
2. Temperature:
   a. May be elevated with bronchopneumonia or heatstroke.
   b. May be depressed by dyspnoeas.
3. Tonsils, pharynx, nose and larynx—any related diseases?
4. Presence of any neoplasm that may have metastasized to lungs?

D. PALPATION

1. Lymph nodes, especially submaxillary:
      Localized or generalized lymphomegaly?
2. Airway:
   a. Larynx (deformities/obstruction/vibration—if noise).
   b. Trachea (collapse/foreign body/injury).
      Palpation may provoke coughing if tracheal irritation is present.
3. Thorax:
   a. Injuries (ribs).
   b. Masses (including the *thoracic inlet* or axillae).
4. Subcutaneous emphysema?
   (with penetrating airway or thoracic wounds).
5. Head or neck oedema? (thoracic mass pressing on venous return).
6. Thickened limbs?
   ('hypertrophic pulmonary osteoarthropathy')
   Secondary to pulmonary or thoracic masses.

E. PERCUSSION

An acquired skill.
1. Increased resonance? (pneumothorax or emphysema).
   (Asymmetry between the two sides?)
2. Regionally decreased resonance?
   (Fluid/masses/pneumonia.)
   (Ruptured diaphragm/pulmonary collapse/oedema.)
3. Horizontal line between resonance and dullness? (effusions).

F. AUSCULTATION

1. *Heart*
   a. Audibility:
      i. Increased by { air/emaciation/anaemia
                        cardiomegaly.
      ii. Muffled by fluids or masses.
   b. Area of cardiac sounds:
      i. Displaced by masses?
      ii. Increased with cardiac enlargement?
   c. Rate (increased in cardiac or respiratory failure).
   d. Rhythm (Chapter 11).
   e. Abnormal sounds (murmurs/gallop rhythms?) (Chapter 12).
2. *Respiratory sounds*
   a. Normal—may be displaced by fluid/mass:
      i. Airway (tracheal or bronchial) harsh/coarse/blowing
         (interrupted to-and-fro).
         Often heard at shoulder level, behind triceps muscle.
      ii. Vesicular (pulmonary alveolar/small bronchi).
          Quiet, soft to-and-fro, rustling sounds.
          Difficult to hear in dogs.
   b. Abnormal:
      i. Wheeze (rhonchi-dry/squeaky/sonorous and continuous)
         (bronchial obstruction—bronchitis/secretions/neoplasia)
         (heard more on expiration than inspiration).
      ii. Crackles—râles (bubbling—alveolar/bronchial fluid)
          —crepitations (partial alveolar collapse)
          (pneumonia/bronchitis/emphysema).
      iii. Pleural friction sounds—when dry inflammation is present
           (to- and-fro squeaks synchronous with respiration).
   N.B. Also auscultate the larynx and trachea:
   locate the precise source of any respiratory noise
   (sounds audible in thorax may be *referred* from elsewhere).

FURTHER READING

O'Brien J. A. (1980) A diagnostic approach to respiratory disease. In: Kirk R. W. (ed.), *Current Veterinary Therapy VII*. Philadelphia, Saunders.

Chapter 7

Further Investigation of Respiratory Disorders

A. THORACIC RADIOGRAPHY

Must be preceded by careful clinical examination.
Very important, because the thoracic cavity is relatively inaccessible.
Relatively more helpful in differentiation of dyspnoeas than coughing.

Indications

    a. To identify/locate/quantify lesions causing respiratory signs.
    b. To identify lesions too small to cause clinical signs.
    c. As a routine check:
        i. For pulmonary metastases in neoplasia.
        ii. Before paracentesis with effusions.
    d. To give a 'quantitative' assessment of progress.

Technique—particular requirements

N.B. Careful handling of dyspnoeic cases is essential.
Good quality films are essential.
    a. At least two views are required (lateral and ventrodorsal)
        —the dorsoventral view is preferred for cardiac outline and for dyspnoeic patients.
    b. The animal must be straight (especially for the ventrodorsal view)—with forelimbs drawn forward to be clear of the chest.
    c. The beam is centred at the caudal edge of the scapula.
    d. Maximum contrast in the lungs is produced at *maximum inspiration* (expiration causes loss of detail/contrast and can

create a false impression of disease although it may occasionally emphasize lesions).

e. Fast exposure times, e.g. 0·01–0·02 sec are desirable to minimize respiratory and cardiac movements—or lungs should be inflated under general anaesthetic.

   Often not obtainable without advanced equipment.

   Aided by the use of extra fast screens and film (e.g. 'rare earth screens').

f. High kV will ensure penetration and reduce time (e.g. 70kV).

g. Grids reduce scatter in deep or broad-chested dogs,
   but require higher exposure factors.

h. Clean screens and careful darkroom technique are essential.

i. A record of exposure factors helps to improve repeated films.

Interpretation

a. Check films for quality—position/exposure/stage of respiration movement.

b. *Systematically* check for shape/size/contour/position/density/ abnormalities:

   i. Bones and extrathoracic structures.
   ii. Diaphragm and thoracic wall.
   iii. Pleural cavity and mediastinum.
   iv. Cardiac outline and size.
   v. Lung fields.
   vi. Airway and bronchi.
   vii. Major blood vessels.
   viii. Oesophagus.

c. Look for:

   i. Displacement of any normal structure (especially by masses/air/fluid/pulmonary collapse).
   ii. Air or other materials in the oesophagus
       (N.B. Air is *common* under general anaesthetic).

d. Examine and identify the *pattern and distribution of any lesions:*

   i. Localize and compare with the other view.
   ii. Determine the site of any lesion:
       Within lung parenchyma?
       Within the mediastinum or pleura?
       Within the airway?

Pattern and distribution of lesions

Often *mixed* patterns—less well-defined than described here.

Often progressive changes (e.g. interstitial → alveolar patterns).

1. Bones and extrathoracic structures

Details:

Fractures, osteomyelitis, neoplasia, swellings, subcutaneous emphysema, liver size, anterior abdominal contents, ascitic fluid?

2. Diaphragm and thoracic wall

Details:

Follow carefully for *integrity:*
acquired ruptured diaphragm is common
(congenital pericardiodiaphragmatic hernias occur rarely).

3. Pleural cavity and mediastinum

Details:

- *a.* Contents: air/fluid/abdominal structures/masses?
  (including lymph nodes).
- *b.* Signs of effusions:
  - i. Air (pneumothorax):
    Elevation of cardiac shadow from the sternum.
    Excessive lucency through much of the thorax.
    Loss of vascular marking of lungs at the periphery of the thorax.
  - ii. Fluid:
    General pleural opacity.
    Loss of detail of the cardiac and diaphragmatic outlines.
    Rounding of lung borders and costophrenic angle.
    Fluid-filled fissure lines between individual lung lobes and between lung lobes and the chest wall.

4. Cardiac outline and size

See Chapter 13.

5. Lung fields

- *a.* *Localized homogeneous lobar disorders* (consolidation):
  Primary lung tumour, large abscess (no air bronchograms), collapse, torsion, haemorrhage.
- *b.* *Alveolar disease* (exudation, bronchiolar occlusion).
  Details:
  - i. Ill-defined, amorphous, fluffy densities, coalescent → blotchy.
  - ii. Air bronchograms (linear/spotty lucent markings) and air alveolargrams → mottling.
  Distribution: Often disseminated and diffuse—in several lobes lobar/segmental distribution—limited by lung borders.

   i. Perihilar in chronic left-sided cardiac failure and some
    granulomatous disorders.
   ii. Cranial and ventral (often patchy)
    in inhalation or broncho-pneumonia.
   iii. Localized to single lobes with haemorrhage.

  Rapid changes often take place (within days or hours);
  densities often blur other details in the lungs.
  c. *Interstitial disease* (fluid/infiltration/fibrosis):
  diffuse densities throughout the lung field
  (resembles uninflated lungs and changes in ageing dogs).
   i. Nodular densities, well-defined (round/irregular/'miliary')
    often at the periphery of lung lobes, visible if > 4 mm
    diameter—with metastatic tumours, granulomatous dis-
    orders, calcification, fibrosis, abscesses.
   ii. Diffuse, unstructured, hazy densities
    —with interstitial pneumonia or haemorrhage.
    (N.B. Severe disease may cause minimal signs.)
   iii. Reticular/linear/honeycombed appearance (unusual)—
    with bronchiectasis, focal fibrosis.

6. *Airway and bronchi*
  a. Few lesions can be seen in the trachea:
   i. Tracheal collapse (only an irregular outline may be seen:
    collapse may be noted only at the time of respiratory
    noise).
   ii. Filaroides nodules (not often visible).
   iii. Haemorrhage (may be seen in coagulopathies).
  b. Bronchial patterns seen within lung fields:
   i. Branching parallel lines and end-on rings—with bronchial
    wall thickening (infiltration/bronchitis/calcification).
   ii. Uneven diameter of bronchi (sacculation > tapering)
    —with bronchiectasis ('bunch of grapes' appearance).
   iii. Occlusion of lumina with exudates, foreign bodies,
    neoplasia.

7. *Vascular changes*
  a. *Hypovascular lungs* (increased lucency):
   i. General:
     Right-to-left shunts (Chapter 13).
     Emphysema.
     Hypovolaemia (shock, dehydration).
     Addison's disease (hypoadrenocorticalism).
   ii. Local: emphysema, blebs, bullae, cysts.
   iii. Artefact—overinflation, overpenetration by X-rays.

    b. Hypervascular lungs/distended vessels
        Left-to-right shunts (Chapter 13).
        Left-sided cardiac failure.
    c. Large, distorted blood vessels
        Angiostrongylus, Dirofilaria.

Other radiographic techniques

    a. Fluoroscopy (screening) can be very useful, especially for airway obstruction, which may vary with respirations.
    b. Positive contrast alimentary studies may be required:
       i. To identify displacement of the oesophagus by masses.
      ii. To identify oesophageal lesions and the integrity of the oesophageal wall.
     iii. To identify abdominal contents in the thorax (with ruptured diaphragm).
  For details *see* p.118
    c. Tomography (layer radiography) for solitary densities
       —can be used to identify the depth and density of a lesion.
    d. Bronchography
      Iodine compounds, tintallum or barium may be used to outline the tracheal and bronchial walls to detect:
       i. Foreign bodies (lucent).
      ii. Lumen damage, bronchiectasis.
     iii. Filling defects (collapse, tumour, Filaroides).
     iv. Displacement by masses.
      v. Lung lobe torsion.
      Under general anaesthesia a little contrast material is poured or blown through a small catheter into the area under investigation.
    e. Angiography—usually assessed with fluoroscopy. Iodinated solutions are introduced by catheter under general anaesthesia (Chapter 13).

B. BRONCHOSCOPY

Strongly indicated in persistent coughing or respiratory noise.
1. For *diagnosis* or confirmation of:
    a. Radiolucent airway foreign bodies.
    b. Tumours:
       i. Intraluminal.
      ii. Pressing on airway.
    c. Filaroides infection.
    d. Tracheobronchitis.
    e. Tracheal collapse.

     f. Tracheal defects or distortion.

     g. Pulmonary exudation (in bronchopneumonia).

2. For *therapy:*

     a. Removal of a foreign body.

     b. Removal of nodules of Filaroides.

     c. (Aspiration of secretion or exudates.)

Equipment

     a. Bronchoscope with distal end lighting.
       A range from 4 mm diam. $\times$ 25 cm long
       to 10 mm diam. $\times$ 50 cm long is required for dogs:

        i. Simple tubes are satisfactory and can be used with alligator forceps and suction if required.

       ii. Sophisticated flexible bronchofibrescopes may be equipped to permit:
            Manipulation of the distal tip.
            Biopsy—with special forceps.
            Suction and aspiration.
            Distal vision.
            Photography

     b. Accessories:

        i. Saline, slides and stains for cytology and to detect parasitic larvae, catheter for flushing.

       ii. Swabs and plates for bacterial culture.

      iii. Suction:
            To aspirate for cytology.
            To clear bronchi.
        But excessive pressure must not be used $\therefore$ a 10-ml syringe is adequate.

      iv. (Laryngoscope and dental mirror for viewing the larynx and pharynx.)

       v. 14-Gauge needle in case of emergency tracheotomy.

Procedure

     a. Equipment must be *sterilized* (chlorhexidine).
       The bronchoscope should be lubricated (KY Jelly).

     b. Anaesthesia following starvation:

        i. Premedication:
            Phenothiazines are desirable.
            Atropine is debatable
            (gives bronchodilatation *but* it thickens secretions).

       ii. Induction—barbiturates intravenously.

      iii. Gas is preferred for maintenance of anaesthesia—to maintain good oxygenation and respiratory control.
      iv. Animal taken to the depth of surgical anaesthesia
        —then anaesthetic is removed during viewing.
      v. Consider muscle relaxants?
  c. The dog is placed in sternal recumbency.
  d. The pharynx and larynx are inspected carefully.
  e. Bronchoscope may be introduced with the aid of a laryngoscope
    —manipulated gently to view:
      i. Mucosa of trachea.
      ii. Tracheal rings and conformation.
      iii. Tracheal bifurcation.
      iv. Main bronchi.

Normal findings

  a. Normal mucosa is pink and glistening
    —blood vessels may be visible.
  b. Tracheal rings are visible through the mucosa
    —the trachea should be round and not distorted.

Abnormal findings

  a. Secretions—may be purulent or haemorrhagic.
  b. Distortion of airway (tracheal collapse).
  c. Hyperaemia/ulceration/roughening of mucosa.

Further investigations

Swabs are taken (via bronchoscope or from the bronchoscope at withdrawal) for culture and sensitivity.
Cytology (saline washing/smear and slide) may reveal:
  a. Malignant cells from primary bronchial neoplasm.
  b. Parasitic larvae (Filaroides/Angiostrongylus).
  c. Leucocytes (bronchopneumonia).
  d. Eosinophils (eosinophilic/allergic pneumonia).
  e. Intracytoplasmic inclusions (distemper).
  f. Bronchial epithelial cells and degeneration (chronic bronchitis).
    (Creighton and Wilkins, 1974.)

C. PARACENTESIS OF THE THORAX

Indicated for pleural effusions and pneumothorax
—for diagnosis and treatment.
  A relatively simple procedure, requiring little equipment.

It is important to *verify* that effusion is present by radiography, and note that an effusion may be localized.

The risk of haemorrhage of pneumothorax is not severe if this technique is carefully applied.

Equipment

    a. 18-gauge needle × 0·75–1 in.
        Or for better results: a plastic cannula with stylette or pleural catheter.
    b. A 3-way tap to assist drainage by allowing removal of syringe without pneumothorax.
    c. Chlorhexidine or similar disinfectant for the skin.
    d. Local anaesthetic.
    e. Syringes and sample bottles (EDTA, heparin and sterile).
    f. (Scalpel blade and suture material.)

Procedure

    a. Area selected: two-thirds way down thorax for fluids; one-third way down thorax for air; 7th or 8th intercostal space; or a local site if indicated radiographically.
    b. The area is clipped and cleaned antiseptically.
    c. Local anaesthetic is infiltrated subcutaneously and into the intercostal space.
    d. (Incision through the skin is advisable if introducing a cannula.)
    e. The animal is restrained in lateral or ventral recumbency.
    f. The needle or cannula is introduced with the 3-way tap attached: at an acute angle to the chest wall to avoid the heart and lungs. Immediately cranial to a rib to avoid vessels and nerve.
    g. A syringe is used to remove fluid.
        If not successful—
        i. Rotate the needle around the whole area.
        ii. Try the other side of the thorax.
        iii. Do not use excessive negative pressure on the syringe.
        iv. May indicate 'pocketing' by adhesions.
    h. Equipment is withdrawn and the skin is sutured if necessary.
    i. The thorax should be re-radiographed.
Stop if pure air, bubbles or clotting fresh blood is withdrawn (may indicate penetration of lung or blood vessel).
    j. Samples should be immediately placed in bottles:
        i. EDTA for cytology.

    ii. Heparin for specific gravity, protein content.
    iii. Sterile bottle for culture and sensitivity.
  k. Smear a sample of fluid on a slide for cytology
     (e.g. using Leishman's stain)
     (spin down → air dry → fix in alcohol → stain for 2–3
     min.).

Nature of effusions

For significance and causes *see* Chapter 3.
  a. True transudate (capillary filtrate):
    Clear, colourless, watery.
    S.G. < 1.015. Total protein < 25 g/l.
    Few cells (< 1000 per c mm).
    (Usually ascites and subcutaneous oedema are also present.)
  b. Modified transudate (raised capillary hydrostatic pressure):
    Yellow/orange/pink, slightly opaque, frothy/fibrin clots.
    S.G. 1.015–1.030. Total protein 25–40 g/l; albumin > globulin.
    Moderate cells (1000–20000 per c mm)
    —mainly RBC, neutrophils and RE cells.
  c. Purulent:
    Cream—green—brown, cloudy/flocculent, often smelly.
    S.G. 1.010–1.030. Total protein 30–60 g/l; globulin > albumin.
    Heavy cells (50000–200000 per c mm)
    mainly neutrophils (often degenerate); numerous bacteria.
  d. Lactescent and chylous*:
    Milky white and opaque; ± blood.
    S.G. 1.015–1.025. Total protein 20–85 g/l; albumin = globulin.
    Moderate/heavy cells (10000–200000 per c mm);
    lymphocytes (pleomorphic) predominate.
  e. Haemorrhagic:
    As true blood, often dark, *rarely clotting* (unless acute).
    S.G. 1.030–1.055. Total protein 40–80 g/l; albumin = globulin.
    Cells much as peripheral blood, but RBC ↓, RE cells ↑.
  f Others:
    i. Neoplastic:
     Variable–orange → haemorrhagic and opaque.
     S.G. 1.013–1.045. Total protein 30–80 g/l;
     albumin = globulin.

---

*To test for true chylous effusion.
    i. Dissolve 5 ml of fluid in 1–2 drops of N NaOH.
    ii. Add equal quantity of ether.
      True chyle should clear.
Also check a smear.
    i. For lymphocytes (neoplastic?)
    ii. For chylomicrons (stain with Sudan III).

Moderate cells (1000–100 000 per c mm).
Some neutrophils and RE cells.
Neoplastic cells may be found (e.g. mesothelioma).
  ii. Bile:
Ochre coloured.
Strongly positive results in tests for *bilirubin.*
S.G. 1.015–1.030. Total protein variable.
Moderate cells (5000–10 000 per c mm).
Neutrophils and RE cells predominate.

Cytology

    a. Inflammatory or neoplastic?
    (N.B. Secondary inflammatory changes are common with bile
    and modified transudates.)
    b. Acute or chronic? (granulocytes → mononuclears with time).
    c. Septic or sterile?
    d. Neoplastic cells present?

D. FURTHER PROCEDURES

1. Biopsy

    a. At thoracotomy—the only way to *confirm* the presence of a
    pleural or pulmonary mass.
    b. With bronchoscopy—sample from an airway lesion to *confirm*
    tumours or parasitic infections.
    c. By needle under general anaesthetic—with lungs inflated,
    using:
        i. A cylindrical cutting needle and an air drill; or
        ii. A Tru-Cut needle (Travenol) (Rosin and Galphin,
            1978).
    Ideally, the needle should be directed with fluoroscopy.
    d. Through the wall of the airway with the forceps of a fibreoptic
    bronchoscope.
Biopsy may be essential to *confirm* a presumptive diagnosis and to
give a prognosis.

2. Thoracotomy

This is necessary:
    a. To examine lesions.
    b. To remove lesions or diseased tissue.
    c. To remove adhesions to allow drainage in exudative pleurisy.
    Procedure requires:
    a. Intermittent positive-pressure ventilation.
    b. Rib resection/retraction.

    c. *Careful* thoracic repair to achieve airtight closure.

    d. Postoperative drainage or Heimlich valve for some cases.

3. Laboratory tests

    a. Routine haematology—of only limited value:

        i. Anaemia is found in haemorrhagic disorders (sometimes also in pyothorax or bronchopneumonia).

        ii. Polycythaemia occurs in some chronic hypoxic disorders.

        iii. Leucocytosis occurs in bronchopneumonia or pyothorax (*uncommon* in tracheobronchitis).

        iv. (Leukaemia is *rare* in lymphosarcoma.)

        v. (Eosinophilia is *not* usually a feature of parasitic infections—but it may occur in some pneumonias.)

    b. Plasma proteins:

        i. Albumin is low in protein-losing disorders.

        ii. Globulins are high in sepsis (pyothorax).

    c. Faecal examination (for Filaroides).

    d. Blood gas analysis.

REFERENCES AND FURTHER READING

Birchard S. J., Cantwell H. D. and Bright R. M. (1982) Lymphangiography and ligation of the canine thoracic duct. A study in normal dogs and three dogs with chylothorax. *J. Am. Anim. Hosp. Assoc.* **18,** 769.

Cantwell H. D. Rebar A. H. and Allen A. R. (1983) Pleural effusion in the dog; principles for diagnosis. *J. Am. Anim. Hosp. Assoc.* **19,** 227.

Creighton S. R. and Wilkins R. J. (1974) Transtracheal aspiration biopsy: technique and cytologic evaluation. *J. Am. Anim. Hosp. Assoc.* **10,** 219.

Creighton S. R. and Wilkins R. J. (1977) Pleural effusions. In: Kirk R. W. (ed). *Current Veterinary Therapy VI.* Philadelphia, Saunders.

Dillon A. R., Pechman R. D., Spano J. S., Teer P. A., Adair S. and Buxton B. (1983) Results of ancillary tests for respiratory disease in normal dogs. *J. Small Anim. Pract.* **24,** 533.

Douglas S. W. and Hall L. W. (1959) Bronchography in the dog. *Vet. Rec.* **71,** 901.

Geary J. C. (1967) Veterinary tomography. *J. Am. Vet. Radiol. Soc.* **8,** 32.

Gibbs C. (1973) Radiological features of intrathoracic neoplasia in the dog and cat. In: Grunsell C. S. G. and Hill F. W. G. (ed.), *Veterinary Annual.* Bristol, Wright Scientechnica.

Lee R. (1976) Pattern of pulmonary disease on thoracic radiographs in dogs and cats. In: Grunsell C. S. G. and Hill F. W. G. (ed.), *Veterinary Annual.* Bristol, Wright Scientechnica.

Lord P. F., Suter P. F., Chan K. F. *et al.* (1972) Pleural, extrapleural and pulmonary lesions in small animals: a radiological approach to differential diagnosis. *J. Am. Vet. Radiol. Soc.* **13,** (2), 4.

O'Brien J. A. and Roszel J. F. (1974) Bronchoscopy and bronchial cytology. In: Kirk R. W. (ed.), *Current Veterinary Therapy V.* Philadelphia, Saunders.

Perman V., Osborne C. A. and Stevens J. B. (1974) Laboratory evaluation of abnormal body fluids. *Vet. Clin. N. Am.* **4**(2), 255.

Rosin E. and Galphin S. P. (1978) Percutaneous drill pulmonary biopsy in the dog. *Am. J. Vet. Res.* **39,** 1547.

Roudebush P., Green P. A. and Digilio K. M. (1981) Percutaneous fine-needle aspiration biopsy of the lung in disseminated pulmonary disease. *J. Am. Anim. Hosp. Assoc.* **17,** 109.

Schall W. D. (1974) Thoracentesis. *Vet. Clin. N. Am.* **4**(2), 395.

Suter P. F. (1980) Interpretation of pulmonary radiographs. In: Kirk R. W. (ed.), *Current Veterinary Therapy VIII.* Philadelphia, Saunders.

Suter P. F. (1984) *Thoracic Radiography. A text atlas of thoracic diseases of the dog and cat.* Wettswil, Switzerland, Suter.

Suter P. F., Carrig C. B., O'Brien T. R. et al. (1974) Radiographic recognition of primary and metastatic pulmonary neoplasms of dogs and cats. *J. Am. Vet. Radiol. Soc.* **15**(2), 3.

Suter P. F. and Lord P. F. (1974) Radiographic differentiation of disseminated pulmonary parenchymal diseases in dogs and cats. *Vet. Clin. N. Am.* **4**(4), 687.

Venker-van Haagen A. J. (1979) Bronchoscopy of the normal and abnormal canine. *J. Am. Anim. Hosp. Assoc.* **15,** 397.

Webbon P. M. and Clarke K. W. (1977) Bronchography in normal dogs. *J. Small Amin. Pract.* **18,** 327.

Chapter 8

Cardiac Disorders

A. COMMON CONGENITAL LESIONS

These represent about 5 per cent of canine cardiac disease (Detweiler and Patterson, 1965).

1. *Causing left-to-right shunts*
    a. Patent ductus arteriosus (PDA).
    b. Ventricular septal defect (VSD).
    c. Atrial septal defects (ASD).
Signs (if not compensated)
Very variable, according to severity and compensation:
    a. (Stunted growth) (especially PDA).
    b. Exercise intolerance and dyspnoea.
    c. Congestive cardiac failure (especially PDA) (Chapter 9).
    d. (May be a *few* signs with septal defects.)

2. *Causing right-to-left shunts*
    a. Tetralogy of Fallot.
    b. Left-to-right shunts with pulmonary hypertension.
    (Usually *serious* defects.)
Signs (if not compensated):
    a. Stunted growth.
    b. Severe exercise intolerance with dyspnoea.
    c. Congestive or right-sided cardiac failure (Chapter 9).

3. *Valvular lesions*
    a. Causing left-sided cardiac failure:
        i. Aortic stenosis.
        ii. Mitral dysplasia/malformation.

Signs (if not compensated):
   i. Exercise intolerance, syncope, dyspnoea, coughing.
   ii. Left-sided cardiac failure (variable) (Chapter 9).
   b. Causing right-sided cardiac failure:
      i. Pulmonic stenosis (very common).
      ii. Tricuspid dysplasia.
Signs (if not compensated)
         Exercise intolerance, dyspnoea, ascites,
         right-sided cardiac failure (Chapter 9).
Breeds most commonly affected (in USA: Patterson, 1971)

PDA	Miniature Poodle Border Collie Pomeranian
Pulmonic stenosis	Chihuahua Beagle* English Bulldog Fox Terrier
Aortic stenosis	Newfoundland* Boxer German Shepherd
Tetralogy of Fallot	Keeshond*

N.B. The incidence may be different in the U.K.,
e.g. pulmonic stenosis may be common in Boxers.

4. *Other congenital cardiovascular anomalies*

   a. Vascular ring strictures (especially persistent right aortic arch)
      i. Cause oesophageal obstruction (Chapter 16).
      ii. Diagnosed with contrast radiology (p. 118).
      iii. Usually no cardiac signs.
   b. Pericardiodiaphragmatic hernia
   Signs
   Variable, may not become apparent for months:
      i. Dyspnoea,
   or ii. Right-sided cardiac failure,
   or iii. Digestive upsets—if intestines involved,
   or iv. An incidental finding.
   Findings
   As for other pericardial disorders—detected radiographically.
   c. Numerous other anomalies have been reported.

---

*Hereditary in some lines (Patterson, 1968).

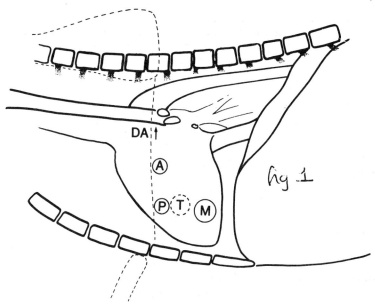

Fig. 1. Sites at which the maximum intensity of murmurs may be located; A, aortic valve; P, pulmonic valve; M, mitral valve; T, tricuspid valve (right-hand side); DA, ductus arteriosus.

General findings with congenital disorders.

Signs (none if heart is compensating)

    a. Cardiac insufficiency, causing weakness or collapse (Chapter 9).

    b. Stunted growth.

    c. Left- or right-sided or congestive cardiac failure (Chapter 9).

Findings

    a. Cyanosis if a right-to-left shunt.

    b. Cardiac *murmurs* (Chapter 12)
    —the site may indicate the source (*Fig.* 1).
    Murmurs are usually *systolic* (*Fig.* 2; p. 80):

    i. Pulmonic or aortic stenosis—the murmur is harsh and well forward (under triceps), centred over the lesion.

    ii. Ventricular septal defect: 'diagonal' murmur, over the left ventricle on the left side and maximal well forward on the right side.

    iii. Mitral and tricuspid dysplasias:
        soft murmurs, centred over the valves.
    iv. Patent ductus arteriosus: 'machinery' murmur, waxing
        and waning through systole and diastole—may be
        localized over base of heart, well forward on the left.
But murmurs may be *absent* in the presence of very large
defects.
  c. Precordial 'thrill'—can be felt at the thoracic wall if the
     vibration of a murmur is sufficient.

Investigations

  a. As for other causes of cardiac failure (Chapters 12 and 13),
     viz:
      i. Try to locate the site and type of the murmur.
     ii. Radiography:
          Undercirculation of lungs with right-to-left shunts.
          Overcirculation of lungs with left-to-right shunts.
          Enlarged right ventricle with: pulmonic stenosis;
          tetralogy of Fallot; most shunts; tricuspid dysplasia.
          Left-sided cardiac enlargement with:
          mitral dysplasia; aortic stenosis.
          Generalized cardiomegaly with patent ductus
          arteriosus.
    iii. ECG—may or may not show diagnostic changes:
          Right axis deviation (negative QRS complex, especially
          lead II)—with pulmonic stenosis, tetralogy of
          Fallot.
          Tachydysrhythmias are common with aortic stenosis.
  b. Cardiac catheterization is required for confirmation:
      i. Angiography (Chapter 13).
     ii. Blood gas analysis if shunts are suspected.
    iii. Blood pressure recordings.

Decisions should be made as to whether:

  a. To return a pup to the breeder.
  b. To warn the client of possible future cardiac failure.
  c. Further diagnostic investigation will indicate prognosis?
  d. Correction is necessary or possible (Chapter 14)?
  e. To breed from the dam or an affected dog—lesions may be
     hereditary.

B. ACQUIRED CARDIAC DISORDERS

These represent 95 per cent of canine cardiac diseases
(Detweiler and Patterson, 1965)

1. Valvular disease

Endocardiosis (valvular fibrosis)

The most frequently encountered heart disease in dogs—the precise cause is unknown. A progressive disease in ageing dogs, especially in small breeds in the UK: Chihuahua, Cavalier King Charles Spaniel, Miniature Poodle, Pekingese.

There is simultaneous deterioration in other tissues (chordae tendineae, etc.) The disease causes progressive valvular incompetence:

    a. The *mitral valve* is most commonly affected.
    Signs:
    Left-sided cardiac failure if heart not compensating eventually progressing to congestive cardiac failure (Chapter 9).
    b. The *tricuspid valve* is also commonly affected, but usually not as severely or predominantly as the mitral valve.
    If primarily affected—causes right-sided cardiac failure (Chapter 9).

General findings

Murmurs— systolic, centred initially over the valve concerned (*Fig.* 1).
    —the duration is short initially, becomes progressively prolonged, the murmur then radiates over the remaining cardiac area.

Treatment

    a. Specific treatment is not available.
    b. Requires management for cardiac failure if this develops (Chapter 14).

N.B. Secondary valvular incompetence often follows cardiac dilatation.

Endocarditis: an uncommon disorder (Lombard & Buergelt, 1983):

Definitive diagnosis is possible with echocardiography, but often made only at post-mortem examination.

Male dogs of large breeds most often affected (aortic valve). Typical agents: Corynebacterium, Erysipelas, Streptococci.

Often, septic (embolic) involvement of other organs occurs (kidneys, CNS, myocardium, joints).

Signs

    a. Those of sepsis: anorexia, lethargy, weight loss.
    b. Involvement of other organs: shifting lameness, painful joints, sign of CNS dysfunction, dyspnoea, epistaxis.
    c. Occasionally congestive cardiac failure.

Findings

    a. Persistent or recurrent pyrexia (variable) and bounding pulse.

    b. Haematuria or pyuria (may be microscopic).

    c. *Changeable* murmur, may be systolic and *diastolic.*

    d. May also be dysrhythmias—if the myocardium is involved.

Investigations

    a. Routine haematology: leucocytosis and often anaemia.

    b. Blood bacterial culture
       —when the dog is pyrexic and *not* receiving antibiotics
       —may be successful only if samples are repeated.

    c. ECG may show tachydysrhythmias or conduction disturbances.

Treatment

    a. Antibiotics (penicillins and/or cephalosporins)
       at high levels, several times daily for several weeks.

    b. Supportive—warmth, rest, attention to feeding.
       —anabolic steroids.

The prognosis is very guarded—embolic spread is common.

2. Myocardial disease

    a. Fibrosis—caused by:
       i. Myocarditis/ischaemia/myocardial dilatation.
       ii. Often secondary to other cardiac disease.

    b. Primary (idiopathic) cardiomyopathy:
       In large and giant breeds of dog. Usually congestive (dilated).

    c. Coronary ateriosclerosis and microscopic infarction:
       i. *Common,* especially in dogs with mitral incompetence.
       ii. May result from cardiac hypertrophy or dilatation.

    d. Myocarditis:
       Septic/immune—mediated/viral (e.g. *Parvovirus*).

    e. Trauma:
       i. Ruptured myocardium causes haemopericardium and acute cardiac failure—can be a sequel to chronic atrial dilatation.
       ii. Contusions (may result in fibrosis).

    f. Infarction—usually caused by:
       i. Septic or neoplastic emboli.
       ii. Intramural coronary arteriosclerosis (*see c. above*).
       (N.B. Atherosclerosis is *rare* in dogs.)

    g. Neoplasms may invade the myocardium:
        i. 'Heart base' tumour (chemodectoma), esp. in Boxers.
        ii. Lymphosarcoma
        or haemangiosarcoma (esp. German Shepherd dogs).
        iii. Other tumour metastases.

Extraneous disorders affecting function (p. 53) include:
    a. Metabolic disorders:
        i. Electrolyte disturbances, esp. potassium and calcium.
        ii. Endocrine disorders, especially thyroid, adrenal.
    b. Toxaemias:
        i. Pyometra, uraemia, hepatic failure, gastric torsion.
        ii. Sepsis.
        iii. Drug toxicity, especially glycosides, anaesthetics.
        iv. Shock (especially, gastric dilatation/torsion).
    c. Hypoxia: especially with respiratory obstruction or
    anaesthesia.

Effects of myocardial disease
    a. Dysrhythmias (Chapter 11).
    b. Loss of myocardial contractility and cardiac output.
This may contribute to:
        i. Cardiac insufficiency (p. 63)
        ii. Congestive cardiac failure.
        iii. Cardiogenic shock (p. 61).

Signs
    a. Left- or right-sided or congestive cardiac failure
    (Chapter 9).
    b. Exercise intolerance, weakness or collapse (Chapter 9).

Findings—can include
    a. *Dysrhythmias* or conduction disturbances (Chapter 11).
    b. Pallor and slow capillary refill.
    c. Weak/rapid/dysrhythmic pulse (Chapter 12).

N.B. It is usually impossible to make a definitive diagnosis of the
underlying myocardial disease *ante mortem.*

Treatment
Usually no specific treatment is available for myocardial disease.
However, the following should be considered:
    a. Treatment for any extraneous disease (see over).

    b. Treatment for any intrinsic disease:
        i. Antibiotics (frequent and prolonged) for myocarditis?
        ii. Corticosteroids for myocarditis?
    c. Treatment for myocardial dysfunction:
        i. Inotropes (glycosides, xanthines) for loss of contractility?
        ii. β blockade (propranolol) for inappropriate hypertrophy.
    b. Specific drugs for dysrhythmias (Chapter 11).
    e. Treatment for congestive cardiac failure (Chapter 14).

3. Pericardial disease

    a. Haemorrhage:
        i. Traumatic (including myocardial rupture).
        ii. Neoplastic (e.g. haemangiosarcoma, 'heart base' tumour).
        iii. Idiopathic/spontaneous (esp. in large dogs).
    b. Transudation—secondary to:
        i. Hypoproteinaemia.
        ii. Venous congestion.
        iii. Venous obstruction (neoplasia).
    c. Exudative pericarditis (uncommon):
        i. Penetrating wounds, foreign body.
        ii. Tuberculosis (now rare).
    d. Fibrinous pericarditis:
        i. Secondary to other disease (autoimmune, uraemic).
        ii. Inflammatory.
Acute dilatation of the pericardial sac is known as 'tamponade'.

Signs
Right-sided cardiac failure (Chapter 9).

Findings

    a. Right-sided cardiac failure—ascites, hepatomegaly, venous congestion.
    b. *Muffled heart sounds,* if effusion is profuse and insidious.
    c. Reduced ECG voltages, sometimes electrical alternans (Tilley, 1985).
    d. Globular cardiac outline on radiographs and sharp edged, if not obscured by effusions (Chapter 13).

Treatment
See Chapter 14.

C. MISCELLANEOUS DISORDERS AFFECTING THE HEART AND CIRCULATION

1. Cor pulmonale

The effect on the heart of respiratory disease, especially where large changes in intrathoracic pressure take place.

Aetiology

    a. Airway obstruction: (Chapter 1):
       (tracheal collapse, chronic bronchitis, laryngeal paralysis)
    b. Severe pulmonary interstitial disease (Chapter 2).
    c. Increased pulmonary vascular resistance.
    d. Pulmonary artery thrombosis or obstruction
       (including dirofilariasis in imported dogs).

Signs

    a. Mainly those of the primary respiratory disease.
    b. Cardiac signs are often minimal.
       But it may cause:
         i. Acute cardiac decompensation.
         ii. Right-sided cardiac failure (Chapter 9).

Findings

    a. Cardiac enlargement (right-sided) on radiographs.
    b. Signs of venous congestion, e.g. hepatomegaly.

2. Metabolic disorders

Hyperkalaemia

Caused by

    a. Hypoadrenocorticalism (Addison's disease) (Chapter 36).
    b. Renal failure (Chapter 28).
    c. Diabetic ketoacidosis (Chapter 36).

Signs

Cardiac insufficiency—weakness, sudden death.

Findings

    a. Bradydysrhythmias—heart blocks, cardiac arrest (Chapter 11).
    b. Microcardia and hypovolaemia may be noted on radiographs.
    c. ECG changes—peaked T wave, suppressed P wave, bradycardia.

Hypokalaemia (uncommon)

Caused by

    a. Gastrointestinal potassium loss.
    b. Urinary loss (especially diuresis).
    c. Excess insulin administration?

Effect

    a. Tachydysrhythmias (Chapter 11).
    b. Depressed T wave on ECG.

Hypocalcaemia

Caused by

    a. Eclampsia.
    b. Hypoparathyroidism (Chapter 36)
    c. Acute pancreatitis.
    d. (Rarely: renal failure, malabsorption).

Effect

    Tachydysrhythmias, excitability.

Hypercalcaemia (*see* p. 212).

Caused by

    a. Hyperparathyroidism
    b. Neoplasia
    c. Hypoadrenocorticalism

Effect

    Bradycardia, weakness.

3. Other extrinsic influences on myocardial function

    a. Hypoxia—caused by:
        Ventilatory, pulmonary disorders, anaesthesia, anaemia, hypovolaemia, congestive cardiac failure.
    b. 'Shock'—involves:
        Endotoxins, myocardial depressant factors, acid-base upsets.
    c. Other organ or system failure (e.g. hepatic or renal).
        General effects—can cause:
        Reduced contractility, dysrhythmias or cardiac arrest.
    d. Obesity:
        i. Increases the work required of the ventricles.
        ii. Restricts pulmonary and cardiac function.

4. Endocrine disturbances (Chapter 36);

  a. Hypothyroidism, diabetes mellitus, hypoadrenocorticalism
  —all reduce myocardial function.
  b. Hyperthyroidism, phaeochromocytoma, hypoparathyroidism
  —all increase myocardial irritability.

5. Functional disturbances (Chapter 11)

  a. Bradydysrhythmias—may reflect excess vagal tone
  —very common in brachycephalic breeds.
  b. Tachydysrhythmias—may reflect excess catecholamines.
  —may be provoked by anaesthesia.

REFERENCES AND FURTHER READING

Atwell R. B. and Kelly W. R. (1980) Canine parvovirus: A cause of chronic myocardial fibrosis and adolescent congestive heart failure. *J. Small Anim. Pract.* **21**, 609.

Darke P. G. G. (1985) Myocardial disease in small animals. *Br. Vet. J.* **141**, 342.

Darke P. G. G. (1986) Congenital heart disease in small animals. *Br. Vet. J.* **142**, 203.

Detweiler D. K. and Patterson D. F. (1965) The prevalence and types of cardiovascular disease in dogs. *Ann. N.Y. Acad. Sci.* **127**, 491.

Ettinger S. J. (1983) Valvular heart disease. In: Ettinger S. J. (ed.), *Textbook of Veterinary Internal Medicine,* 2nd ed. Philadelphia, Saunders.

Ettinger S. J. and Suter P. F. (1970) *Canine Cardiology.* Philadelphia, Saunders.

Feldman E. C. (1980) Influence of non-cardiac disease on the heart. In: Kirk R. W. (ed.), *Current Veterinary Therapy VII.* Philadelphia, Saunders.

Gibbs C., Gaskell C. J., Darke P. G. G. et al. (1982) Idiopathic pericardial haemorrhage in dogs: a report of 14 cases. *J. Small Anim. Pract.* **23**, 483.

Gooding J. P., Robinson W. F., Wyburn R. S. et al. (1982) A cardiomyopathy in the English Cocker Spaniel: a clinico-pathological investigation. *J. Small Anim. Pract.* **23**, 133.

Harris S. G. (1971) Some problems of the pericardium. *J. Am. Anim. Hosp. Assoc.* **7**, 27.

Hayes H. M. (1975) An hypothesis for the aetiology of canine chemoreceptor system neoplasms, based on an epidemiological study of 73 cases among hospital patients. *J. Small Anim. Pract.* **16**, 337.

Hayes M. A., Russell R. G. and Babiuk L. A. (1979) Sudden death in young dogs with myocarditis caused by parovirus. *J. Am. Vet. Med. Assoc.* **174**, 1197.

Liu S-K., Maron B. J. and Tilley L. P. (1979) Canine hypertrophic cardiomyopathy. *J. Am. Vet. Med. Assoc.* **174**, 708.

Lombard C. W. (1984) Echocardiographic and clinical signs of canine dilated cardiomyopathy. *J. Small Anim. Pract.* **25**, 59.

Lombard C. W. and Buergelt C. D. (1983) Vegetative bacterial endocarditis in dogs; echocardiographic diagnosis and clinical signs. *J. Small Anim. Pract.* **24**, 325.

Murdoch D. B. and Baker J. B. (1977) Bacterial endocarditis in the dog. *J. Small Anim. Pract.* **18**, 687.

Patterson D. F. (1968) Epidemiological and genetic studies of congenital heart disease in the dog. *Circulat. Res.* **23**, 171.

Patterson D. F. (1971) Canine congenital heart disease: epidemiology and etiological hypotheses. *J. Small Anim. Pract.* **12,** 263.

Pearson G. R. and Head K. W. (1976) Malignant haemangioendothelioma (angiosarcoma) in the dog. *J. Small Anim. Pract.* **17,** 737.

Shouse C. L. and Meier H. (1956) Acute vegetative endocarditis in the dog and cat. *J. Am. Vet. Med. Assoc.* **129,** 278.

Sisson D. and Thomas W. P. (1984) Endocarditis of the aortic valve in the dog. *J. Am. Vet. Med. Assoc.* **184,** 570.

Thomas W. P., Reed J. R., Baver T. G. and Breznock E. M. (1984) Constrictive pericardial disease in the dog. *J. Am. Vet. Med. Assoc.* **184,** 546.

Tilley L. P. (1985) *Essentials of Canine and Feline Electrocardiography.* Philadelphia, Lea & Febiger.

Tilley L. P., Liu S-K. and Fox P. R. (1983) Myocardial disease. In: Ettinger J. (ed.) *Textbook of Veterinary Internal Medicine.* (2nd Ed). Philadelphia, Saunders.

Chapter 9

Cardiac Failure

The presence of cardiac disease is easily detected (Chapter 12). However, much cardiac disease may not be very relevant in pet dogs. Signs of cardiac *failure* and compensation must therefore be assessed. The heart and circulation have great powers of *compensation* for disease and falling output, especially if slow in onset.

Mechanisms of compensation

a. Peripheral vasoconstriction—increases the circulating volume.
b. Tachycardia.
c. Increased myocardial contractility
   (and subsequent myocardial hypertrophy).
d. Cardiac chamber enlargement → stroke volume increase.
   Increased venous return (*a*) → stroke volume increase.
e. Decreased renal perfusion leads to stimulation of:
   aldosterone ∴ sodium and fluid retained
   → plasma volume increase.
   angiotensin → peripheral vasoconstriction.

These mechanisms may be *inappropriately regulated* in congestive cardiac failure, causing:

a. Excessive tachycardia.
b. Excessive vasoconstriction and afterload.
c. Volume overload.
d. Myocardial hypoxia.

Decompensation is provoked by

a. Myocardial disease or hypoxia → { loss of contractility.
                                    { dysrhythmias.

    b. Increased valvular incompetence, especially if the heart
        dilates.
    c. Excess demands on the heart:
       i. Obesity.
      ii. Excessive activity and exercise.
     iii. Excessive heat or humidity.
     iv. Pregnancy.

Acute decompensation may be precipitated by:
    a. Pericardial effusion (haemorrhage → tamponade).
    b. Rupture of chordae tendineae.
    c. Acute myocardial failure.
    d. Development of severe dysrhythmias.
    e. Respiratory diseases.
    f. Renal failure.
    g. Fluid therapy.
    h. Shock, haemorrhage, trauma.
    i. Toxaemia or sepsis.
    j. Anaemia.

N.B. Cardiac failure rarely induced by anaesthesia *per se,* but
anaesthetic *hypoxia* may provoke fatal dysrhythmias.

Failure to compensate

This can cause one of the following clinical syndromes:
    a. Left-sided cardiac failure.
    b. Right-sided cardiac failure.
    c. Congestive cardiac failure (left-sided and right-sided).
    d. Acute left ventricular failure (cardiogenic shock).
    e. Cardiac insufficiency.

A. LEFT-SIDED CARDIAC FAILURE

Aetiology
    a. Congenital aortic stenosis.
    b. Congenital mitral dysplasia.
    c. Mitral incompetence (endocardiosis).
    d. Cardiomyopathy (especially large dogs).
    e. Aortic outflow obstruction.
    f. (Dysrhythmias.)

Failure to compensate results in

Pulmonary congestion and oedema, causing:

Either—Four stages in the development of *chronic* left-sided cardiac
       failure, as defined by Ettinger and Suter (1970):

Stage   I—Normal activity does not produce undue fatigue, dyspnoea or coughing.

II—The dog is comfortable at rest, but ordinary activity causes fatigue, dyspnoea or coughing.

III—The dog is comfortable at rest, but minimal exercise may produce fatigue, dyspnoea or coughing. Signs may also develop when the dog is recumbent.

IV—Congestive heart failure: dyspnoea and coughing are present even at rest.

Signs are exaggerated by any physical activity.

Or — Signs of *acute* decompensation (uncommon):
a. Sudden and severe dyspnoea.
b. 'Air hunger', respiratory noise.
c. Coughing of frothy material.
d. (Sternal recumbency.)

Findings

Assess signs of compensation/decompensation:
a. Cyanosis—rare unless severe pulmonary oedema.
b. Weak pulse (variable).
c. (May be hepatomegaly if also venous congestion.)
d. Auscultation—associations with cardiac failure:
   i. Increased area over which cardiac sounds may be heard.
   ii. Tachycardia is usually present.
   iii. Gallop rhythms (presence of S_3, S_4)—(Chapter 12).
   iv. *Murmurs*—with congenital or valvular disease.
   v. *Dysrhythmias*—with associated myocardial disease.
   vi. Pulmonary râles.

Coughing and dyspnoea must be differentiated from other causes (Chapter 5), as a murmur of mitral incompetence may be an incidental compensated finding in the presence of other significant respiratory disease.

Investigations

a. Look for evidence of cardiac compensation/decompensation (Chapter 12):
   i. Cardiac enlargement (auscultation and radiographs).
   ii. Tachycardia and loss of sinus arrhythmia.
   iii. Weakened pulse.

    b. Radiography (*Figs.* 3, 4) (Chapter 13).
    c. Electrocardiography:
        i. For dysrhythmias.
        ii. Indicating chamber enlargement?
    d. Reduced pVO_2 (<35 mmHg)?

B. RIGHT-SIDED CARDIAC FAILURE

Aetiology

    a. Congenital pulmonic stenosis.
    b. Congenital tricuspid dysplasia.
    c. Tricuspid incompetence (endocardiosis).
    d. Congestive cardiomyopathy (esp. in large dogs).
    e. Pericardial effusions.
    f. Neoplasia ('heart base' tumour).
    g. Cor pulmonale.
    h. Dirofilariasis (imported dogs).
    i. Other myocardial disorders.
    j. Secondary to left-sided failure.

Failure to compensate results in

    a. Venous congestion.
    b. Hepatomegaly, splenomegaly.
    c. Ascites.
    d. Hydrothorax—variable.
    e. (Occasionally: ventral subcutaneous oedema.)

Signs

    a. Abdominal distension (ascites).
    b. Exercise intolerance.
    c. Dyspnoea (especially if pleural effusion).
    d. (Subcutaneous oedema—uncommon.)

Findings

    a. (Venous congestion.)
    b. Ascites (Chapter 34).
    c. Hydrothorax (Chapter 3).
    d. Hepato- and splenomegaly—often palpable.
    e. ± Muffled heart sounds (pleural and/or pericardial effusions).
    f. Murmurs—in most cases.
    g. Dysrhythmias—in many cases.

Investigations

    a. Radiography (*Figs.* 5, 6, pp. 86, 87).
    b. Paracentesis of thorax or abdomen
        —*modified transudate* (Chapter 7).
    c. Electrocardiography:
        i. Dysrhythmias? (Chapter 11).
        ii. Cardiac chamber enlargement?
    d. Pericardiocentesis—if evidence of pericardial effusion
        (Chapter 14).
    e. Raised central venous pressure? (> 10 cm water).

C. CONGESTIVE CARDIAC FAILURE

This includes signs of simultaneous failure of both left and right sides. However, neither side is in isolation and a degree of failure of both sides is often present especially in volume overload.

Aetiology

    a. Left-to-right shunts, including:
        i. Patent ductus arteriosus.
        ii. (Ventricular septal defect.)
    b. Myocardial failure.
    c. Sequel to left- or right-sided failure.

Signs

    a. Lethargy, exercise intolerance, weight loss.
    b. Dyspnoea.
    c. Coughing.
    d. Abdominal distension.

Findings

    a. Usually a weak, rapid pulse.
    b. Often dysrhythmias.
    c. Usually murmurs.

D. ACUTE LEFT VENTRICULAR FAILURE
(Cardiogenic shock—reduced cardiac output)

Aetiology

    a. Reduced ventricular filling:
        i. Cardiac tamponade (pericardial effusion).

    ii. Obstruction of the caudal vena cava
       (especially if a dog is placed in dorsal recumbency) by:
          Abdominal mass (Chapter 34).
          Gastric dilatation (Chapter 17).
          Uterus—gravid or metritis.
    iii. Tension pneumothorax.
    iv. Hypertrophic cardiomyopathy.
     v. Excessive ventricular hypertrophy.
    vi. Intracardiac neoplasia.
  b. Reduced ventricular emptying, especially with *reduced contractility.*
      May also cause pulmonary oedema.
     i. Acute cardiac decompensation (*see* p. 59).
    ii. Dysrhythmias of sudden onset.
    iii. Congestive cardiomyopathy—giant breeds of dog.
    iv. Myocardial, hypoxia/ischaemia.
     v. Myocardial toxins, anaesthetics.
    vi. Obstruction of left ventricular outflow.
Circulatory shock may also be due to:
  a. Neural causes (vasomotor tone ↓ → venous return ↓).
  b. Sepsis → fall in vasomotor tone.
  c. Anaphylaxis/endotoxins.
  d. Hypotensive drugs.
  e. Hypovolaemia/haemorrhage.
  f. Myocardial depressant factors (in 'shock')

Signs

Lethargy/weakness/collapse.

Findings

  a. Pallor of mucous membranes.
  b. Very slow capillary refill.
  c. Weak or absent pulse.
  d. Reduced intensity of cardiac sounds?
  e. Tachycardia.
  f. Cardiac dysrhythmias?
  g. Radiographic signs of venous congestion or cardiac failure?
  h. Raised central venous pressure (> 10 cm water) unless hypovolaemic.

Treatment

  a. Cage rest ± oxygen therapy?
  b. Treat dysrhythmias or cardiac arrest (Chapters 11 & 15).

    c. Intravenous fluid therapy
    d. Positive inotrope? (dopamine 10–20 μg/kg/min in drip or isoprenaline).

E. CARDIAC INSUFFICIENCY (output failure; 'heart attack')

Episodes of fainting, collapse, ataxia or gross exercise intolerance may be due to cerebral hypoxia resulting from poor cardiac output. This is especially likely to occur with sudden increases in demand, and with anaemia or respiratory hypoxia.

Aetiology

    a. Acquired mitral incompetence.
    b. Congenital subaortic (or pulmonic) stenosis.
    c. Congenital shunts.
    d. Myocardial disease → { poor contractility / dysrhythmias
    e. Functional disturbances (dysrhythmias).
    f. Other causes of acute left ventricular failure (D).
(N.B. Massive coronary atherosclerosis and myocardial infarction are *rare* in dogs.)

Signs

    a. Occurrence with excitement or exercise.
    b. Lack of prodromal or post-ictal signs.
    c. The animal is usually flaccid while collapsed.
    d. Usually weakness or unconsciousness.
    e. Very rapid recovery with minimal distress.

Findings

Left-sided or congestive cardiac failure?
Dysrhythmias (Chapter 11) especially: bradycardias (< 60 beats/min); multiple extrasystoles; paroxysmal tachycardias (> 180 beats/min).
Murmurs (congenital disorder or acquired mitral incompetence).
    N.B. Cyanosis is uncommon in cardiac failure (p. 68) except with:
    a. Right-to-left shunts.
    b. Severe pulmonary oedema

Management

For dysrhythmias—*see* Chapter 11.

Exercise may need to be controlled, as cardiac output cannot readily be increased: this form of cardiac failure is not easily treated.

DIFFERENTIAL DIAGNOSIS OF SUBCUTANEOUS OEDEMA

1. Generalized oedema

    a. Hypoproteinaemia:
        i. Nephrotic syndrome (p. 167)
        ii. Protein-losing enteropathy (p. 128)
        iii. (Hepatic failure/starvation)—uncommon.
    b. Right-sided or congestive cardiac failure.
    c. Hypoaldosteronism.

2. Localized oedema

    a. Venous or lymphatic obstruction:
        neoplasia/thrombosis/inflammation/F.B.
    b. Allergic reaction/insect sting.
    c. Burns/lymphangitis.
    d. Arteriovenous fistula (shunt).

Investigation

Check the heart, pulses, plasma proteins (hypoalbuminaemia?). Radiograph to check for any obstructing mass.

REFERENCES AND FURTHER READING

Bown P. (1974) Oedema in the dog. In Grunsell C.S.G. and Hill F.W.G. (Eds.) *The Veterinary Annual,* 19th Ed. Bristol, Scientechnica.
Ettinger S. J. and Suter P. F. (1970) *Canine Cardiology.* Philadelphia, Saunders.
Fisher E. W. (1967) Cardiac failure. *J. Small Anim. Pract.* **8,** 137.
Pensinger R. R. (1971) Congestive heart failure in dogs. *J. Am. Vet. Med. Assoc.* **158,** 447.

Chapter 10

Differential Diagnosis of Episodic Weakness or Collapse

Many non-cardiac causes of weakness or collapse exist, in addition to cardiac insufficiency.

1. CNS hypoxia

    a. Cardiac insufficiency (*see* p. 63).
    b. Airway obstruction, severe coughing (Chapter 1).
    c. Anaemias, methaemoglobinaemia, haemorrhage (Chapter 42)
    d. Vascular occlusion/vasospasm/thrombosis.
    e. Arteriovenous fistulae.
    f. Vasomotor/vasovagal syncope (especially in brachycephalics?).
    g. Ventilatory disorders (pleural, pulmonary, airway).

2. Functional CNS disorders

    a. Primary epilepsy.
    b. Narcolepsy (instantaneous falling asleep).

3. Metabolic disorders affecting the CNS/heart/peripheral muscles

    a. Hypoglycaemia (Chapter 36):
        i. Pancreatic islet cell tumour/other neoplasms.
        ii. (Hypoadrenocorticalism.)
        iii. (Hepatic failure/storage diseases.)
        iv. (Idiopathic.)
    b. Hyperkalaemia (Chapter 36):
        i. Hypoadrenocorticalism (Addison's disease.)

    ii. (Renal failure.)
    iii. Diabetic ketoacidosis.
  c. Hypocalcaemia (Chapter 36):
    i. Lactation tetany ('eclampsia').
    ii. Acute pancreatitis.
    iii. (Hypoparathyroidism.)
    iv. (Hypoproteinaemia/malabsorption.)
  d. Hyperammonaemia (hepatic failure) (Chapter 24):
    i. Congenital portosystemic shunts.
    ii. Hepatic cirrhosis or neoplasia.
  e. Uraemia (terminal renal failure) (Chapter 28).
  f. Other disturbances (including hyponatraemia, hypokalaemia).
  g. Poisons (heavy metals/insecticides/glycol).
  h. Neoplasia, chronic sepsis.

4. Primary upper CNS lesions

  a. Congenital (e.g. hydrocephalus or storage diseases).
  b. Encephalitis
    (distemper/rabies/toxoplasma/louping ill/Aujeszky's disease).
  c. Neoplasia.
  d. Otitis media/interna.
  e. Trauma.
  f. Haemorrhage.
  g. Meningitis.

5. Spinal/orthopaedic/neuromuscular disorders

  a. Congenital spinal disorders:
    (e.g. dysraphia, wobblers or vertebral malformations).
  b. Bilateral limb (e.g. luxated hips) or spinal trauma.
  c. Acquired spinal disorders:
    Prolapsed intervertebral disc/trauma/tumour/CDRM.
  d. Neuromuscular and muscular disorders:
    Myasthenia gravis/botulism/cramp/azoturia/
    polymyositis/tetanus/myotonia.
  e. Peripheral nerves:
    Brachial plexus neuritis/polyneuritis/lumbo-sacral
    neuropathy.

6. Psychogenic/idiopathic syncope

Many dogs 'faint' recurrently for no apparent cause.

It is important to relate to clients so that they appreciate that episodes of collapse are common and usually not fatal.

DIAGNOSTIC PROCEDURE FOR COLLAPSE

History

A client should be very carefully questioned to establish the pattern and precise nature of the collapse/seizure.

Very important to establish (figures and letters refer to previous section):

    a. *The pattern*—whether:
   i. Collapse is episodic (1*a*,*b*; 2*a*,*b*; 3*a*,*b*; 4*a*,*b*,*g*; 6).
   ii. There is continuing weakness (1*c*,*d*,*e*; 3*b*,*d*,*e*; 4*c*,*d*,*e*,*f*; 5).
   iii. Previous episodes?—and their character, duration, pattern.

    b. *The circumstances* of the collapse—whether:
   i. At exercise or with excitement (1*a*,*b*,*c*,*e*; 2*b*; 3*a*,*b*,*c*; 5*d*).
   ii. At rest or on waking (2*a*).
   iii. Associated with feeding or starvation (3*a*,*d*).

    c. Whether *prodromal signs* occur? (2*a*; 3?).

    d. *Consciousness*—is the dog:
   i. Conscious when collapsed? (5; sometimes 1; 3; 4).
   ii. Unconscious when collapsed? (2; 6; often 1).

    e. The *activity* when the dog is collapsed—whether:
   i. Flaccid (1; 2*b*; 5; 6; sometimes 3).
   ii. Tonic-clonic spasm (2*a*; sometimes 3; 4*a*,*b*,*g*; 5*d*).

    f. The *behaviour on recovery* from collapse—is there:
   i. Rapid and instantaneous recovery? (1*a*,*b*; 2*b*; 6).
   ii. Post-ictal bewilderment? (2*a*; 3?; 4?).
   iii. Continuing weakness? (1*c*,*d*,*e*; 3; 5).

    g. The *exercise tolerance*—whether it is:
   i. Generally good (2; 6).
   ii. Generally poor (1; 3; 4; 5).

    h. The dog's *general behaviour* at other times.
   (Are there CNS signs, generalized metabolic disease?).

    i. The *dog's age*—for example:
   i. Young dogs (1*a*?; 2; 3*c*;*d*?; 4*a*; 5*a*).
   ii. Ageing dogs (1*d*; 3*a*,*e*,*h*; 4*c*; 5*c*).

Findings

    a. Generalized illness (toxaemias, metabolic disorders)?
    b. Other CNS signs?
   (check facial expression, eyes, cranial, spinal reflexes).
    c. Mucous membranes: pallor or cyanosis? (Ask the client.)

    d. Check for the presence of any cardiac *disease*:
        i. Dysrhythmias—but may be transient.
       ii. Murmur? (congenital or acquired).

Further investigations

    a. Routine haematology: anaemia?
    b. Blood urea/glucose/Na^+/K^+/Ca^{2+}/ammonia/lead?
    c. Liver enzyme levels/CPK?
    d. ECG, EEG?
    e. Radiology?—spine/heart/liver/skull? (usually unhelpful).

DIFFERENTIAL DIAGNOSIS OF CYANOSIS

(Due to an excess of circulating reduced haemoglobin) (> 50 g/l):
1. Cardiovascular disorders:
    a. Right-to-left shunts (Chapter 8).
    b. Pulmonary arteriovenous shunts.
    c. Pulmonary thrombosis.
    d. (Pulmonary oedema.)
2. Airway obstruction (Chapter 1).
3. Pulmonary disorders (Chapter 2):
    a. Interstitial diseases (e.g. viral pneumonia or paraquat
       poisoning).
    b. Alveolar diseases (e.g. oedema or bronchopneumonia).
4. Pleural cavity disorders (Chapter 3).
    Effusions or masses, ruptured diaphragm.
5. Haemoglobin deficiencies:
    Methaemoglobinaemia
    (enzyme deficiency, or nitrite or chlorate poisoning).
6. Delayed or impaired tissue perfusion ('shock').

Investigations

    a. Thoracic radiography:
       To check for respiratory or pleural disorder.
    b. Haematology:
       To check for methaemoglobinaemia or compensatory poly-
       cythaemia in long-standing cases.
    c. May require cardiac catheterization (Chapter 13) for:
        i. Angiography
       ii. Blood gas analysis (arterial samples).

FURTHER READING

Beckett S. D., Branch C. E. and Robertson B. T. (1978) Syncopal attacks and sudden death in dogs: mechanisms and etiologies. *J. Am. Anim. Hosp. Assoc.* **14**, 378.

Farrow B. R. H. (1980) Episodic weakness. In: Kirk R. W. (ed.), *Current Veterinary Therapy VII.* Philadelphia, Saunders.

Holliday T. A. (1980) Seizure disorders. *Vet. Clin. N. Am.* **10**, 3.

Mitler M. M., Soave O. and Dement W. C. (1976) Narcolepsy in seven dogs. *J. Am. Vet. Med. Assoc.* **168**, 1036.

Chapter 11

Cardiac Rhythm and Dysrhythmias

All cardiac tissue has intrinsic rhythmicity:
1. The sinus node is the *dominant pacemaker.*
2. Sites in the ventricular conduction tissue may act as *substitute pacemakers* (especially bundles of His/Purkinje system)—if there is no stimulus from above (due to blocks or sinus arrest).
   This usually produces bradycardia with 'escape' beats.
In addition:
3. Myocardial lesions may act as irritant foci creating *ectopic pacemakers* which will precede the normal activation from the sinus node if premature.

NORMAL RHYTHMS

1. **Sinus rhythm** represents normal regular activation of the atria, and via the conduction system, the ventricles by the pacemaker (sinus node) at a normal rate.
2. **Sinus 'arrhythmia'** is very common in normal dogs.
   (Regular phasic acceleration and deceleration in heart rate—often synchronous with respirations.)
   a. Usually a sign of a well-compensating heart.
   b. May be accentuated in respiratory disease or airway obstruction.
   c. Usually no gross change in P wave shape on ECG.
   d. Usually abolished with tachycardia.
3. **Sinus tachycardia.** Regular rhythm of sinus node origin at rates of 150–200/min.
   Significance
   a. Physiological—exercise/fear/stress/pyrexia/toxaemia/anaemia.

70

b. Pathological—response to cardiac failure.
Important to identify the source of rhythm by ECG.
ECG: normal P-QRS-T wave form—at a fast rate.
Therapy:
May respond to digitalization or beta blockade if excessive.

DYSRHYTHMIAS

DIAGNOSIS OF DYSRHYTHMIAS

a. Auscultation—attention should be paid to:
   i. Intensity of sounds.
   ii. Pattern of rhythm.
   iii. Comparison of cardiac rhythm with the pulse.
b. Electrocardiography (*see* Tilley, 1985).
   Reflects myocardial events and impulse conduction *only*.
   Does not diagnose:
   i. Valvular or congenital lesions.
   ii. Loss of myocardial contractility.

N.B.:
a. Diagnosis of a dysrhythmia does not necessarily indicate the precise aetiology.
b. Dysrhythmias *per se* may or may not necessarily contribute significantly to cardiac failure.

1. Bradydysrhythmias

a. Conduction disturbances, caused by:
   i. Excess vagal tone.
   ii. Myocardial lesions (abscesses/fibrosis/neoplasms) invading the conduction tissue.
b. Myocardial or pacemaker depression by:
   toxaemias/electrolyte disturbances/glycosides.

Sinus arrest/pause

a. Long pauses between groups of beats.
b. May be synchronous with respirations.
c. May be an accentuation of sinus arrhythmia:
   i. Common in brachycephalic dogs.
   ii. Similar pause occurs in the pulse.
   iii. Of significance if prolonged (may cause syncope).
   iv. Occasional ventricular escape beats may occur.
d. May be abolished with atropine if vagal in origin.

'Missed' or 'dropped' beats

Absence of one or more beats in normal sequence
—with a simultaneously dropped pulse.
ECG: absence of:
- *a.* P-QRS-T if sino-atrial block.
- or *b.* QRS-T if atrioventricular block.
  Of limited significance unless frequent.
  May be abolished with atropine if vagal in origin.

Bradycardia (Heart rate less than 60/min)

- *a.* If notably regular, it may indicate *complete heart block*
  —the pulse may be notably strong.
  - i. *ECG:* P waves totally dissociated from QRS and T
    but waveforms may be of normal shape.
  - ii. Usually a slow ventricular *escape* rhythm.
  - iii. May be serious: neoplasia/toxaemia/metabolic upset.
  - iv. May cause syncope or congestive cardiac failure.
- *b.* If any regularity in the grouping of beats is present, the rhythm
  may be sinus arrhythmia or sinus bradycardia.
- *c.* It may represent hyperkalaemia (Addison's disease or toxaemia):
  Reduced P waves on ECG, and QRS-T waveform changes.

Severe bradycardia may cause cardiac insufficiency or congestive
cardiac failure.

Ventricular arrest/standstill

Represents *cardiac arrest* (Chapter 15).

2. Tachydysrhythmias

Ectopic irritant foci (caused by myocardial disease or irritability) may
intervene or replace the dominant pacemaker if premature.
Producing:
- *a.* Atrial or ventricular premature beats.
- *b.* Atrial (or ventricular) fibrillation.
- *c.* Paroxysmal atrial or ventricular tachycardias.

Exacerbated by:
- *a.* Hypoxia/acidosis/hypothermia/catecholamines/
  hypocalcaemia.
- *b.* Depression of normal pacemaker.

Ectopic beats (atrial or ventricular premature beats)

Heard as premature and louder beats ('tripping' in a tachycardia).
There may be a pulse deficit ⎫
Any murmur may be altered ⎭ for the beat.

ECG:
    a. If an atrial ectopic beat there may be:
        i. Prematurity or apparent absence of P wave.
        ii. P waveform change.
        iii. Prematurity of QRS (with slight voltage change).
or *b.* If a ventricular ectopic beat:
        i. Prematurity of QRS with bizarre shape.
        ii. Increased duration of QRS.
        iii. Absence of associated P wave.
    Ectopic beats are a common finding in cardiac failure.
    Usually represent myocardial disease or irritability (Chapter 9).
    May contribute to cardiac failure.
Therapy—no treatment is necessary unless very frequent:
    a. Withdraw any cardiac glycosides.
    b. Consider:
        i. lignocaine i.v. in emergency.
        ii. quinidine, disopyramide, β blockade or tocainide.

Atrial fibrillation or flutter

True arrhythmia—'tumultuous' heart.
Random variations in rhythm, intensity of sounds and any murmurs.
Pulse deficit and variability in strength of the pulse.
ECG:
    a. Absence of P waves, usually 'f' waves present.
    b. Random irregularity of QRS complexes.
    c. Variations in QRS and T voltages.
More common in large and giant breeds than in small dogs.
Serious—usually associated with severe myocardial disease; usually
associated with congestive cardiac failure.
Therapy for atrial fibrillation:
    a. Digitalization may help by reducing the ventricular rate.
    b. β blockade will usually reduce the ventricular rate.
    c. (Quinidine is rarely effective in dogs in reversing fibrillation.)
But
    d. DC current shock is occasionally effective (Ettinger, 1968).

Paroxysmal tachycardias (atrial or ventricular)

Continuous or intermittent bursts of tachycardia with a regular rhythm
and rate of > 200/min.
Usually a rapid and weak pulse.
ECG:
    a. P waves may (atrial) or may not (ventricular tachycardia) be
        present.
    b. QRS-T may be of bizarre waveform if ventricular tachycardia.

Usually represents severe myocardial disease.

May cause weakness or syncope.

May respond to β blockade, quinidine or lignocaine.

Ventricular fibrillation

Represents *cardiac arrest* (Chapter 15).

THERAPY FOR DYSRHYTHMIAS

1. Bradydysrhythmias

Principles

        Check for any extrinsic systemic disease.

        Treat any reversible myocardial disease.

        Attempt to reverse any vagal hyperactivity.

        Increase the heart rate.

        Withdraw cardiac glycosides if in use.

   a. *Atropine*—blocks vagal hyperactivity.

     Indications:

       i. Heart blocks.

       ii. Sinus arrest.

       iii. Sinus bradycardias.

     Contraindication: Tachycardias.

     Dosage: 0·6–2·0 mg by injection i.v., s.c.

           0·5–2·0 mg orally every 8 hours.

   b. *Isoprenaline* (Saventrine; Pharmax) (β adrenergic stimulant).

     Indications:

       i. Sinus arrest.

       ii. Sinus bradycardias.

       iii. Total atrioventricular block.

     Contraindication: Tachydysrhythmias.

     Dosage: 15–30 mg t.d.s. orally.

     N.B. Use with *care*—occasionally this drug may cause sudden death (due to ventricular fibrillation?)

   c. *Artificial pacemakers.*

     Indications: cardiac inefficiency associated with:

       i. Sinus arrest or bradycardia.

       ii. Total atrioventricular block.

     Application:

       i. Requires a ventricular pacemaker and lead.

       ii. The lead is placed directly into the epicardium (transthoracic/abdominal) or via great veins into the right ventricle.

       iii. The pacemaker is placed subcutaneously, e.g. at the neck. Stability may be improved by use of a Dacron pouch.

       iv. Requires careful supervision and follow-up.

2. Tachydysrhythmias

Principles

Check for any extrinsic systemic disease (p. 53).
Treat any reversible myocardial disease (p. 50).
Reduce myocardial irritability.
Suppress substitute pacemakers and automaticity.

    a. Lignocaine (without adrenaline) (Xylocard; Astra).
      Indications:
        i. Paroxysmal ventricular tachycardia.
        ii. Ventricular fibrillation.
        iii. Multiple ventricular premature beats.
      For *acute* dysrhythmias.
      Contraindication: Heart blocks.
      Dosage: 2–5 mg/kg of 2 per cent *slowly* i.v.
          or 50–120 µg/kg/min in drip
          (as it is excreted within 30 minutes)
      Toxicity: depression/muscle tremors/convulsions can occur.

    b. Quinidine sulphate
      Indications:
        i. Atrial flutter or fibrillation—but rarely reversible in dogs.
        ii. Paroxysmal atrial or ventricular tachycardia.
        iii. Multiple ventricular ectopic beats.
      Contraindications:
        i. Decompensated congestive cardiac failure
          (it decreases myocardial contractility).
        ii. Heart blocks.
      Dosage: 6–10 mg/kg every 4–8 hours orally.
      Toxicity: depression, anorexia, vomiting, diarrhoea, convulsions, heart block, cardiac arrest.

    c. Procainamide
      Similar application to quinidine.
      125–500 mg every 4–6 hours orally.

    d. β *blockade,* e.g. propranolol (Inderal; ICI)
      Indications: supraventricular tachydysrhythmias:
        i. Paroxysmal atrial tachycardia.
        ii. Atrial fibrillation—to lower the ventricular rate.
        iii. Hypertrophic/obstructive myocardial disorders—to reduce myocardial work and oxygen consumption.

Contraindications:

i. Care should be taken in congestive cardiac failure, as myocardial contractility and circulatory preload are reduced.

ii. Bradydysrhythmias.

Dosage: 0·05 mg/kg by slow i.v. injection.

0·1–1·0 mg/kg every 8 hours orally.

e. Disopyramide (Rythmodan: Roussel)

Increases the refractory period and slows Purkinje conduction.
Indications: similar to those of quinidine, especially ectopic pacemakers. (May be less toxic than quinidine.)
Dosage: 50–200 mg t.d.s. (capsules).

f. Tocainide (Tonocard; Astra)

Oral form of lignocaine—a new drug.
Dosage: 30 mg/kg t.i.d. orally.
Toxicity: vomiting, convulsions.

REFERENCES AND FURTHER READING

Bohn F. K., Patterson D. F. and Pyle R. L. (1972) Atrial fibrillation in dogs. *Br. Vet. J.* **127**, 485.

Darke P. G. G., Been M. and Marks A. (1985) Use of a programmable, 'physiological' cardiac pacemaker in a dog with total atrioventricular block. *J. Small Anim. Pract.* **26**, 295.

Ettinger S. J. (1968) Conversion of spontaneous atrial fibrillation in dogs, using direct current synchronized shock. *J. Am. Vet. Med. Assoc.* **152**, 41.

Ettinger S. J. (1983) Cardiac arrhythmias. In: Ettinger S. J. (ed.), *Textbook of Veterinary Internal Medicine*, 2nd Ed. Philadelphia, Saunders.

Hilwig R. W. (1976) Cardiac arrhythmias in the dog: detection and treatment. *J. Am. Vet. Med. Assoc.* **169**, 789.

Lombard C. W., Tilley L. P. and Yoshioka M. (1981) Pacemaker implantation in the dog: survey and literature review. *J. Am. Anim. Hosp. Assoc.* **17**, 751.

Macintire D. K. and Snider T. G. (1984) Cardiac arrhythmias associated with multiple trauma in dogs. *J. Am. Vet. Med. Assoc.* **184**, 541.

Muir W. W. and Lipowitz A. J. (1978) Cardiac arrhythmias associated with gastric dilatation—volvulus in the dog. *J. Am. Vet. Med. Assoc.* **172**, 683.

Patterson D. F., Detweiler D. K., Hubben K. et al. (1961) Spontaneous abnormal cardiac arrhythmias and conduction disturbances in the dog. *Am. J. Vet. Res.* **22**, 355.

Tilley L. P. (1985) *Essentials of Canine and Feline Electrocardiography*. Philadelphia, Lea & Febiger.

Yoshioka M. M., Tilley L. P., Harvey H. J. et al. (1981) Permanent pacemaker implantation in the dog. *J. Am. Anim. Hosp. Assoc.* **17**, 746.

Chapter 12

Investigation of Cardiac Disease

The presence of cardiac *disease* is readily detected by auscultation. The diagnosis of cardiac *failure* may also be aided by careful clinical assessment.

HISTORY AND OBSERVATIONS

See Chapter 9.
(N.B. History and signs may be minimal if cardiac disease is *compensated.*)

PALPATION

1. Pulse (femoral artery)
Not as valuable in dogs as might be anticipated.

Pulse quality
Depends on:
    a. Arterial pressure:
        i. Myocardial contractility.
        ii. Blood viscosity.
    b. Peripheral vascular resistance:
        i. Capillary constriction/dilatation.
        ii. Arteriovenous shunts.
    c. Palpability—varies with:
        i. Hindlimb conformation.
        ii. Physical condition of the dog.

Pulse character

    a. Strong/full/firm (easy to feel):
        i. Excitement or exercise.
        ii. Myocardial hypertrophy.
        iii. Renal fibrosis.
    b. Soft/weak (readily compressed):
        i. (Mitral incompetence.)
        ii. Aortic stenosis.
        iii. Myocardial failure.
        iv. Paroxysmal tachycardias.
        v. Peripheral vasodilatation or shunt.
    c. Thready/empty:
        i. Anaemia or hypoproteinaemia.
        ii. Terminal illness.
        iii. Myocardial failure.
    d. 'Water-hammer' (rapid collapse):
        Left-to-right shunts.
    e. Absence:
        i. Iliac thrombosis.
        ii. Neoplastic obstruction.
        iii. Cardiac arrest.
    f. Variable intensity: (usually with dysrhythmias):
        i. Atrial fibrillation.
        ii. Ventricular premature beats.
        iii. Heart blocks.

Pulse Rate

Normal dog: 70–140 per minute.
Affected by physiological processes, psychology and behaviour:
    a. Rapid:
        i. Paroxysmal tachycardias (*see* Chapter 11),
            Cardiac failure).
        ii. Reflex tachycardias with:
            Activity/excitement.
            Shock/anaemia.
            Fever/pain.
    b. Slow: bradydysrhythmia, CNS depression.
N.B. Compare with the heart rate for *pulse deficit.*
This is common in dysrhythmias:
e.g. atrial fibrillation/ventricular premature beats.

Pulse rhythm

Regular (sinus rhythm) or sinus arrhythmia is normal.
Auscultation is more valuable for accessing rhythm (Chapter 11).

Pulse pressure

May be recorded:
- *a.* Directly (carotid/femoral/ear artery).
- *b.* Indirectly (limb or tail)—with cuff and oscillometry.

But diagnostic information is not readily obtained in dogs.

2. Apex beat

Reflects movement of the myocardium.
Often prominent with cardiac enlargement and in thin-skinned or narrow-chested breeds.
Can be recorded (Apexcardiography—Scott-Park, 1986).

3. Precordial thrill

Vibrations of a severe, harsh murmur may be *felt*,
especially with aortic or pulmonic stenosis or septal defects.

PERCUSSION

1. *May* indicate an enlarged area of cardiac dullness—but not very helpful in dogs.
2. May be dullness in ventral thorax with pleural effusions—in right-sided or congestive cardiac failure.

AUSCULTATION OF CARDIAC SOUNDS

1. **Audibility**/intensity of sounds/area over which heard:
   - *a.* Increased by:
     - i. Cardiac enlargement.
     - ii. Anaemia/fever.
     - iii. Emaciation.
     - iv. Pneumothorax.
   - *b.* Decreased by:
     - i. Pleural effusion or mass.
     - ii. Pericardial effusion.
     - iii. Obesity or heavy coat.
     - iv. (Addison's disease or toxaemia.)
   - *c.* Displaced by masses in the thorax.

2. **Heart rate** (*see* Pulse):
   - *a.* Generally increased in cardiac failure (and with fear/fever/excitement/exercise).
   - *b.* Decreased in some dysrhythmias (Chapter 11).

3. Rhythm (*see* Chapter 11, Dysrhythmias).

4. Abnormal sounds
   a. Murmurs are vibrations due to turbulence of blood—caused by:
      i. Changes in plasma or blood viscosity
         (e.g. anaemia or hypoproteinaemia).
      ii. Lesions in the blood flow-path (congenital or acquired): shunts/stenotic lesions/valvular incompetence.
      iii. Cardiac dilatation (in heart failure).
   Fortunately, nearly all turbulence is at audible frequencies.
   b. Friction sounds.
      May occur synchronously with the heart beat,
      e.g. pericardial adhesions or pleural adhesions.
   c. 'False' murmurs are also heard.
      May vary with the stage of respiration; with the heartrate; and from day to day.
      (Often airway sounds being influenced by the heart beat.)
   d. Gallop rhythms—often indicate cardiac failure:
      i. Due to accentuation of sounds (especially if atrial overload):
         Third heart sound (ventricular filling—S_3; *Fig.* 2).
         Fourth heart sound (atrial contraction—S_4; *Fig.* 2).
      ii. Due to duplication of the second sound (S_2; *Fig.* 2) if:
         Dilatation of a ventricle.
         Delay in closure of pulmonic/aortic valve.

Murmurs may be described:
   a. By *site:* centre of maximum intensity and distribution
      (may indicate origin/valve) (*Fig.* 1, p.47).
   b. By *intensity*—may be graded:
      I. Faintest audible murmur—not immediately heard on auscultation.
      II. Faint, but heard within a few seconds.
      III. Immediately audible (and widespread).
      IV. Loud murmur audible even with the chest piece not quite in contact with the thorax.
      V. Very loud murmur, audible even with the chest piece slightly withdrawn from the thoracic wall.
   (The grade *may* be associated with the severity of the lesion.)
   c. By *pitch/frequency/*character, e.g.:
      i. Soft, blowing (e.g. mitral incompetence).
      ii. Harsh, crescendo—decrescendo (e.g. pulmonic stenosis).
      iii. Squeaky (friction—pericardial rubs).
      iv. High-pitched or musical (sometimes mitral incompetence).

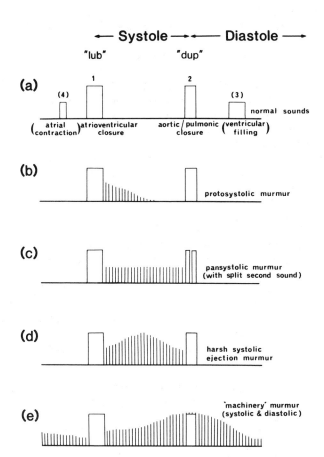

Fig. 2. Heart sounds and murmurs (*a*) Normal sounds: S3 and S4 are not normally audible in dogs (except sometimes in heart failure). S1 and S2 are not necessarily caused *by* valve closure. (*b*) Protosystolic murur, as in early mitral incompetence. (*c*) Pansystolic murmur, as in advanced mitral incompetence. S2 is often inaudible. Splitting of S2 (as shown) is occasionally found in ventricular enlargement. (*d*) Systolic ejection murmur, as in congenital pulmonic or aortic stenosis. (*e*) 'Machinery' murmur that waxes and wanes throughout systole and diastole, as in patent ductus arteriosus.

(Indicates the type of lesion.)
  d. By *phase of the cardiac cycle* (*Fig.* 2):
        i. Murmurs are usually *systolic,* as they are created by high
             pressures.
       ii. Diastolic murmurs are uncommon in dogs.
             They are usually found in association with systolic
             murmurs, e.g. in endocarditis, where they change character
             rapidly, or with patent ductus arteriosus—a continuous,
             but varying 'machinery' murmur.
This description is aided by phonocardiography (Chapter 13).

5. Other findings

Râles and rhonchi are commonly found in pulmonary oedema—with left-
sided or congestive cardiac failure (Chapter 9).

REFERENCES AND FURTHER READING

Detweiler D. K. and Patterson D. F. (1967) Abnormal heart sounds and murmurs of the
    dog. *J. Small Anim. Pract.* **8,** 193.
Gay C. C., McCarthy M., Carter J. et al. (1978) Relationship between apex cardiogram
    and left ventricular pressure events in Greyhound dogs. *Am. J. Vet. Res.* **39,** 1322.
Scott-Park F. M. (1986) Quantitative assessment of cardiac function in dogs, using the
    apexcardiogram. Edinburgh University, PhD Thesis.

Chapter 13

Further Investigation of Cardiac Disease

Cardiac radiology is of more value than other simple aids in the assessment of cardiac failure. ECGs are primarily indicated in dysrhythmias.

A. CARDIAC RADIOLOGY

Cardiac radiology indicates cardiac enlargement, circulating volume and signs of congestive cardiac failure (very useful).

The general principles are as for thoracic radiography (Chapter 7) *but:*
1. The dorsoventral view is preferred to ventrodorsal for the cardiac outline.
2. The beam must be centred over the heart—level with the caudal corner of the scapula.
3. Anterior abdominal details are valuable and should be included.

Examine films for—

  a. Overall cardiac size (depends on chest shape)—normally:
    i. On the lateral projection:
     Craniocaudally: 2½–3½ rib spaces
     (increased in right-sided and congestive failure).
     Dorsoventrally: less than three-quarters the depth of the thorax (increased in left-sided failure).
     The distal trachea is parallel to the sternum in normal dogs.
    ii. On the dorsoventral projection:
     Laterally: less than two-thirds the width of the thorax.

But these measurements are very variable.

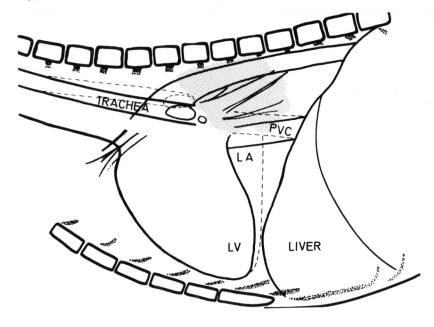

Fig. 3. Diagram of a lateral view of the thorax, showing changes found in left-sided cardiac failure.----- indicates displacement of structures; shading indicates typical site of pulmonary oedema. LA, left atrial enlargement; LV, left ventricle; PVC, caudal (posterior) vena cava.

   b. *Individual cardiac chamber enlargement* (*Figs.* 3–6):
      i. Left atrial enlargement:
           Elevation of the trachea.
           Straightening of the caudal border of the heart.
           Elevation of the caudal vena cava.
      ii. Right-sided: the heart lies cranially along sternum.
      iii. The apex may be displaced by enlarged ventricles on the dorsoventral film—to the left or to the right.
   c. Effects of *left-sided cardiac failure* on pulmonary tissues:
      i. Chronic failure typically → *perihilar* oedema.
      ii. Acute failure often → *generalized* alveolar density.
      iii. Vascular congestion—dilated vessels.
   d. Signs of *right-sided* or congestive cardiac failure:
      i. Pleural cavity effusion.
      ii. Enlargement of caudal vena cava.
      iii. Enlarged liver and/or ascites.

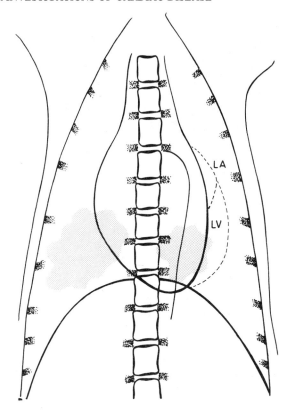

Fig. 4. Diagram of a dorsoventral view of the thorax, showing changes found in left-sided cardiac failure. ----- indicates enlarged structures; shading indicates typical sites for pulmonary oedema. LA, left atrial enlargement; LV, left ventricular enlargement.

e. *Other findings,* e.g.:
   Pulmonary hypovascularity with:
      i. Hypovolaemia.
      ii. Right-to-left shunts.
      iii. Hypoadrenocorticalism.
Angiography may be essential to confirm the presence of congenital lesions:
      i. Selective—by cardiac catheterization.
      ii. Non-selective—via a needle into:
            The jugular vein.
            The left ventricle.

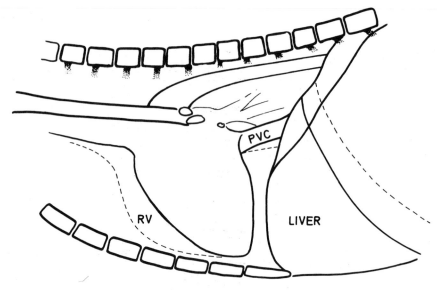

Fig. 5. Diagram of a lateral view of the thorax, showing changes found in right-sided cardiac failure. ----- indicates enlarged structures. RV, right ventricular enlargement; PVC, enlarging caudal (posterior) vena cava.

Using iodine solutions (e.g. Conray 420; May & Baker) (p. 88).

Fluoroscopy (with an image intensifier) is valuable:
    i. In angiography.
    ii. In the diagnosis of pericardial effusions.

B. ELECTROCARDIOGRAPHY

This records:
1. Heart rate.
2. Cardiac rhythm and impulse conduction.
3. Waveform—which may be influenced by:
    a. Cardiac chamber enlargement.
    b. Myocardial function and metabolism.

ECGs in no way indicate *cardiac output*—they can be almost normal in an animal dying of cardiac failure.

For the *technique* and interpretation: *see* Tilley (1985).

Important:

ECG artefacts are common unless care is taken to:
1. Ensure good electrode contact with the skin.

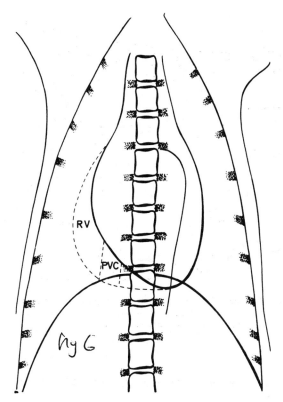

Fig. 6. Diagram of a dorsoventral view of the thorax, showing changes found in right-sided cardiac failure. ----- indicates enlarged structures. RV, right ventricular enlargement; PVC, enlarging caudal (posterior) vena cava.

   a. Clip hair, spirit the skin?
   b. Use *plenty* of electrode jelly, *rubbed in* well.
2. Ensure dry feet and coat and use an insulated floor or table.
3. Minimize movement—allow the dog to *relax*
   without shaking/panting/moving about.
   Place a small dog in a basket?

C. PHONOCARDIOGRAPHY

Many electrocardiographs can also record cardiac sound waves synchronously with the ECG.

This may help to identify:
1. The relationship of murmurs to the normal cardiac sounds.
2. The duration of murmurs.
3. The frequency (pitch) and form of murmurs.

D. CARDIAC CATHETERIZATION

Essential for *confirmation* of the presence of intracardiac
or vascular lesions by:
1. Selective angiography:
   Radio-opaque iodine compounds (e.g. Conray 420; May & Baker)
   (1 ml/kg body weight) are introduced by rapid injection.
   The flow is recorded by one of these techniques:
   a. Rapid X-ray cassette changer (2 films/sec).
   b. Cineradiographic film.
   c. Fluoroscopy and video tape.
2. Intracavity blood pressures, e.g. pressures are elevated in:
   a. The left ventricle in aortic stenosis (also *low* in the aorta).
   b. The right ventricle in:
      i. Pulmonic stenosis (also low in the pulmonary artery).
      ii. Ventricular septal defect.
      iii. Tetralogy of Fallot.
   c. The right atrium in atrial septal defect.
3. Blood gas analysis (Ettinger and Suter, 1970):
   a. Over-oxygenation is found in right ventricle and/or pulmonary
   artery samples in left-to-right shunts.
   b. Hypoxic samples are obtained from the aorta with right-to-left
   shunts
   (also with respiratory disease and cyanotic disorders, p. 68).
   c. Excessive carbon dioxide content is found in pulmonary
   disorders (Chapter 2).
   d. Venous oxygen is reduced in cardiac failure.
4. Central venous pressure is elevated (> 10 cm H_2O) in venous
   congestion.

Also essential if cardiac output studies are contemplated.

Technique

(Under general anaesthesia and with asepsis.)
Ideal catheter sizes: 6 or 7 French gauge.
   a. Left-sided catheterization:
      i. Easiest via the carotid artery—but requires dissection;
      more difficult to enter the left ventricle from the femoral
      artery.

  ii. Repeated *gentle* urging will allow the catheter through the aortic valve when open.

  iii. Difficult to enter the left atrium with conventional catheters.

 b. Right-sided catheterization:

  i. Easily achieved via the jugular vein.

  ii. Passes into the right atrium, then the right ventricle.

  iii. Pulmonary arterial 'wedge' pressure can also be recorded.

E. LABORATORY TESTS

Few specifically diagnostic tests are available.

The following observations may be made in cardiac failure:

1. Routine haematology:
   a. Mild anaemia and leucocytosis common in congestive failure.
   b. Gross neutrophilia with a left shift occurs in endocarditis.
   c. Polycythaemia with right-to-left shunts.
2. Blood urea:
   Slight elevation (to twice normal) is common in congestive failure.
3. Liver enzyme levels:
   Slight elevation is common in congestive or right-sided failure.
4. Plasma proteins:
   There is a tendency for protein levels to fall, especially globulin.
5. Muscle enzymes:
   CPK and LDH may be elevated in acute myocardial disease.
6. Venous oxygen (pVO_2) depressed (< 35 mmHg) in congestive failure.

F. OTHER TECHNIQUES

There is no simple test for cardiac failure, myocardial contractility, or ventricular volume overload.

Various techniques are under development which may prove helpful.

1. Echocardiography

Use of ultrasonic scan to assess the depth, volume and function of tissues (especially the myocardium).

Useful in diagnosis of volume overload, myocardial activity, valvular motion, pericardial effusions.

A technique with great potential for the future.

2. Apexcardiography

(recording the movements created by the cardiac apex)

Produces a waveform from which an assessment of myocardial contractility and systolic time intervals may be derived.

3. Cardiac imaging

Radioisotopes are now used in man in conjunction with gamma radiation cameras to identify areas of myocardial disease. Useful in man for discovering areas of ischaemia resulting from infarction.

REFERENCES AND FURTHER READING

Bolton G. R. (1975) *Handbook of Canine Electrocardiography*. Philadelphia, Saunders.

Bonagura J. D., Myer C. W. and Pensinger R. R. (1982) Angiocardiography. *Vet. Clin. N. Am.* **12**(2), 239.

Bonagura J. D. and Pipers F. S. (1981) Echocardiographic features of pericardial effusions in dogs. *J. Am. Vet. Med. Assoc.* **179**, 49.

Bonagura J. D. and Pipers F. S. (1983) Diagnosis of cardiac lesions by contrast echocardiography. *J. Am. Vet. Med. Assoc.* **182**, 595.

Buchanan J. W. and Patterson D. F. (1965) Selective angiography and angiocardiography in dogs with congenital cardiovascular disease. *J. Am. Vet. Radiol. Soc.* **6**, 21.

Darke P. G. G. (1974) The interpretation of electrocardiograms in small animals. *J. Small Anim. Pract.* **15**, 537.

Ettinger S. J. and Suter P. F. (1970) *Canine Cardiology*. Philadelphia, Saunders.

Gay C. C., McCarthy M., Carter J. et al. (1978) Relationship between apex cardiogram and left ventricular pressure events in Greyhound dogs. *Am. J. Vet. Res.* **39**, 1322.

Lombard C. W. (1984) Echocardiographic and clinical signs of canine dilated cardiomyopathy. *J. Small Anim. Pract.* **25**, 59.

Myer C. W. and Bonagura J. D. (1982) Survey radiography of the heart. *Vet. Clin. N. Am.* **12**(2), 213.

Pipers F. S., Andrysco R. M. and Hamlin R. L. (1978) A totally non-invasive method for obtaining systolic time intervals in the dog. *Am. J. Vet. Res.* **39**, 1822.

Pipers F. S., Bonagura J. D., Hamlin R. L. and Kittleson M. (1981) Echocardiographic abnormalities of the mitral valve associated with left-side heart disease in the dog. *J. Am. Vet. Med. Assoc.* **179**, 580.

Suter P. F. and Lord P. F. (1971) A critical evaluation of the radiographic findings in canine cardiovascular diseases. *J. Am. Vet. Med. Assoc.* **158**, 358.

Tilley L. P. (1985) *Essentials of Canine and Feline Electrocardiography*. Philadelphia, Lea & Febiger.

Wyburn R. S. and Lawson D. D. (1967) Simple radiography as an aid to the diagnosis of heart disease in the dog. *J. Small Anim. Pract.* **8**, 163.

Chapter 14

Management of Cardiac Failure

Few cardiac lesions can be cured; management of chronic heart disease is therefore important.

The intensity of therapeutic measures depends on the stage of development of failure, especially following mitral incompetence (Chapter 9).

GENERAL APPROACH

1. Correct or reduce underlying disease or dysfunction.
   Not applicable in many cases:
   - *a.* Surgical correction of congenital defects.
   - *b.* Paracentesis of pericardial effusions.
   - *c.* Therapy for dysrhythmias (Chapter 11).
   - *d.* Therapy for infections in myocarditis or endocarditis.
2. Reduce demands on the heart:
   - *a.* Exercise restriction (p. 93).
   - *b.* Dietary restriction in obesity.
   - *c.* Prevention of pregnancy.
   - *d.* Sedation? if there is severe coughing or excitement.
3. Relieve circulatory overload in congestive failure:
   - *a.* Diuresis (reduces pre-load).
   - *b.* Salt-free diet.
   - *c.* Peripheral vasodilatation:
     - i. Arteriolar (hydralazine):
       Reduces afterload
       Increases cardiac output
     - ii. Ateriolar and venous (prazosin, captopril);
       Reduce preload and afterload.

4. Improve myocardial contractility, e.g. in congestive cardiomyopathy:
    a. Cardiac glycosides.
    b. Xanthine derivatives.
5. Reduce myocardial work, irritability and oxygen consumption:
    β blockade (also reduces after-load).
6. Further symptomatic therapy:
    a. Bronchodilation? (xanthines)—most helpful in coughing.
    b. Removal of pleural effusion/ascites:
    paracentesis (*see* Chapters 7 and 34).
    If affecting respirations or if not effectively relieved by diuresis.
    c. Oxygen in severe heart failure with dyspnoea?
7. Careful advice and instruction to the client and frequent patient monitoring are very important in cardiac management.

DETAILS OF CARDIAC THERAPY

1. Surgical correction of congenital defects

    a. Ligation of vascular lesions (vascular ring strictures, patent ductus arteriosus). *Relatively* simple—following thoracotomy, the vessel should be double-ligated with silk, and sectioned. Ductus can recanalize if not thoroughly occluded.
    b. Corrections not requiring cardiac bypass:
      i. Pulmonic stenosis *can* be relieved by right ventricular puncture and opening the constriction.
      ii. Pericardio-diaphragmatic hernia can be reduced.
    c. Corrections requiring cardiac bypass ('heart–lung machine'). Very sophisticated equipment and a surgical team are required. It is *possible* but expensive to repair most defects, e.g. aortic stenosis, septal defects, tetralogy of Fallot, dysplastic valves.

Corrections should generally be carried out as early as possible, following treatment for any congestive failure.

2. Paracentesis for pericardial effusions

    a. Approach similar to thoracentesis (Chapter 7):
    asepsis, local analgesia, small incision.
    b. Site: 5th right intercostal space, two-thirds way down thorax.
    c. Needle: 2–3 in × 16 g over-the-needle or through-needle cannula;
    also need a 3-way tap and syringe.
    d. Technique:
      i. The cannula and needle are advanced across the thorax.

ii. The pericardium is usually felt scratching the needle. It is then punctured.

iii. The needle is removed, replaced immediately by syringe.

iv. Fluid is withdrawn as necessary, using 3-way tap, through the cannula.

The patient should be monitored by ECG—ectopic (premature) beats may indicate accidental myocardial penetration.

If fluid is haemorrhagic—check for clotting (intracardiac blood should clot, pericardial blood usually does not).

If haemorrhage recurs, consider partial pericardectomy.

3. Exercise restriction

This is very important in cardiac failure. Any exercise/activity/excitement may require output beyond the reserves of compensation:

a. Discourage: hill- and stair-climbing, stick or ball-chasing, long walks at the first signs of failure (fatigue/dyspnoea/cough).

b. Limit dogs to lead exercise.

c. Cage rest with no exercise is essential in severe failure.

4. Diuresis

Very important in the volume overload of congestive failure.

Advantages

Counteracts the retention of sodium and water (volume overload). Relieves the effects of:

a. Pulmonary congestion/oedema.

b. Ascites/hydrothorax/venous congestion.

Disadvantages

Hypotension, loss of cardiac output and hypovolaemia *may* occur. Loss of potassium can occur at high dose rates.

Frusemide and thiazides

a. Are potent and very rapid in action.

b. Can be used in combination with other therapy.

c. Are relatively non-toxic and safe but can cause dehydration.

d. The dose may be adjusted to effect.

e. Potassium loss may be significant at high doses and either (i) potassium supplementation (Slow K) or (ii) spironolactone (Aldactone) (10–50 mg orally t.d.s.) is worth consideration, but these add expense and can equally be overdosed.

f. Should be used cautiously if renal dysfunction is present.

    g. May be used at higher than recommended dosage in severe cardiac failure, but cardiac output may fall.

Normal dose for frusemide:

    a. Acute failure: 1–2 mg/kg body weight b.d. or t.d.s.

    b. Chronic failure: 1–4 mg/kg body weight *once* daily to effect.

5. Salt-free diet

Excess dietary sodium creates an unnecessary excretory load for the circulation in cardiac failure and intake should be limited. The following should be *avoided* if possible:

    a. Most commercial foods (tinned, dried, biscuits, meal) and prepared meats and bread, as these usually contain added salt.

    b. Eggs, milk and milk products and fish, as these have a high sodium content.

Advise clients to cook meat for the animal, with pasta, potatoes or rice as a source of carbohydrate. Vegetables may be fed as required. Poor palatibility can reduce the acceptance of salt-free foods—frying the food or the use of sodium-free savourings may be tried.

6. Peripheral vasodilators

    a. Arteriolar dilators reduce after-load in cardiac failure:
        i. Improve tissue perfusion.
        ii. Reduce ventricular overload and mitral incompetence.
        iii. Increase cardiac output.

Effective in *terminal* cardiac failure—but may be temporary. e.g. hydralazine (Apresoline: Ciba) at 0·5–2·0 mg/kg b.d. orally.

    b. Combined arteriolar and venodilators also reduce preload— useful in volume overload (congestive or left-sided failure):
        i. Prazosin (Hypovase; Pfizer) at 0·02–0·05 mg/kg b.d. orally.
        ii. Captopril (Capoten; Squibb) at 0·1–1·0 mg/kg t.d. orally.
        This is also antagonistic to angiotensin and aldosterone.
        May cause marrow depression and thrombocytopenia?

N.B. Any vasodilator can cause weakness or collapse—*use with care.*

7. Digitalization

Cardiac glycosides are widely used, but often misused.
Digoxin is preferred to digitoxin, and as a well-standardized product (e.g. Lanoxin tablets or Lanoxin PG Elixir; Wellcome).

Objectives
- a. To improve myocardial contractility.
- b. To slow inefficient tachycardia.
- c. To prolong diastole—potentially improves ventricular filling and coronary perfusion.

Disadvantages
- a. Increased oxygen demand by myocardium?
- b. Prolonged conduction of impulse ⎫ which can
- c. Increased myocardial irritability ⎭ provoke dysrhythmias.
- d. Narrow therapeutic margin—readily toxic.
- e. Of doubtful efficacy in many cases.

Indications
- a. Atrial fibrillation—to control the ventricular rate.
- b. To control atrial tachycardias.
- c. To increase contractility in congestive cardiomyopathy?

Contraindications
- a. Certain dysrhythmias:
  - i. Heart blocks.
  - ii. Ventricular premature (ectopic) beats.
  - iii. Paroxysmal ventricular tachycardia.
- b. Systemic illness or signs of toxicity;
  (depression, anorexia, gastrointestinal disturbance).
- c. Excessive myocardial hypertrophy (e.g. aortic stenosis).

Dosage

No fixed dose—each application must be a trial. Ideally, a plasma level of 1–2 μg/l indicates adequate therapy, if it can be measured (De Rick et al., 1978).

Administration
- a. *Rapid intravenous:*
  - i. Now rarely used.
  - ii. Diuresis is safer and more rapid in effect.
- b. *Moderately rapid* (oral)—best applied to kennelled dogs:
  A total *loading dose* of 0·05–0·20 mg/kg body weight is calculated and given in divided doses over 48 hours until:
  - i. Signs of toxicity of any dysrhythmia are noted.
  - ii. Signs of effectiveness (lowered heart rate or increased P-Q interval on ECG).
  - iii. Adequate plasma levels (2μg/l) can be demonstrated.

Therapy should then cease for at least 24 hours, and resumed at a daily oral dose of ¼ to 1/10 of the loading dose that was required.

    c. Slow oral digitalization can be employed in outpatients: 0·02 mg/kg body weight/day in divided doses (slightly less if Elixir)to a maximum of 0·75 mg/kg/day—increased if necessary after 1 week.

Notes

    a. Animals receiving glycosides must be checked regularly for bradycardia or dysrhythmias.

    b. Clients should be warned to stop administration if in any doubt about the animal's well-being.

    c. Old dogs, puppies and giant breeds need relatively less drug.

8. Xanthine derivatives

Aminophylline, theophylline, etamphylline are widely used, but these agents are *not* very potent.

Advantages

    a. Mild diuresis.
    b. Bronchodilatation.
    c. Increased myocardial contractility.
    d. Relatively inexpensive and safe.
    e. Can be used with other agents.

Disadvantages

    a. Increased myocardial demand for oxygen.
    b. May increase dysrhythmias.

Most helpful for coughing in early stages of left-sided failure and for intravenous use in acute cardiac failure.

9. Sedation

Barbiturates and opiates (e.g. morphine 0·2–0·5 mg/kg s.c.) are relatively safe for use in congestive cardiac failure for excitable animals, for distress or where coughing (especially nocturnally) poses problems.

TREATMENT OF ACUTE CARDIAC FAILURE

Acute decompensation of left-sided cardiac failure produces severe pulmonary oedema (Chapter 9), requiring rapid and potent therapy:

1. Cage rest.
2. Intravenous diuresis, e.g. frusemide (2–5 mg/kg body weight)—results may be noticeable within 15 min.

3. Intravenous xanthine derivatives: given slowly.
4. Suction (small polythene tube and syringe)
   and posture (lower the head)—to clear the airway.
5. Oxygen therapy?—but a mask is often not well tolerated by a distressed dog.
6. Morphine (0·2–0·5 mg/kg body weight, s.c., t.d.s.).
7. Vasodilator therapy may give relief:
   a. Sodium nitroprusside (Nipride; Roche) 5–20 μg/kg/min i.v.
   b. ? Hydralazine (Apresoline; Ciba) 5–20 mg slowly i.v.
8. Antidysrhythmic therapy may be necessary (Chapter 11).
9. Cardiac inotrope?–dopamine (10 μg/kg/min in drip).
10. Other therapies (now rarely necessary):
    a. Phlebotomy.
    b. Intravenous glycosides.

REFERENCES AND FURTHER READING

Darke P. G. G. (1984) Therapy for cardiac failure in small animals. *Vet. Rec.* **115,** 329.

Davis L. E. (1980) Pharmacodynamics of digitalis, diuretics and antiarrhythmic drugs. In: Kirk R. W. (ed.). *Current Veterinary Therapy VII.* Philadelphia, Saunders.

De Rick A., Belpaire F. M., Bogaert M. G. et al. (1978) Plasma concentrations of digoxin and digitoxin during digitalization of healthy dogs with cardiac failure. *Am. J. Vet. Res.* **39,** 811.

Detweiler D. K. and Knight D. H. (1977) Congestive heart failure in dogs: Therapeutic concepts. *J. Am. Vet. Med. Assoc.* **171,** 106.

Ettinger S. J. (1966) Therapeutic digitalization of the dog in congestive heart failure. *J. Am. Vet. Med. Assoc.* **148,** 525.

Ettinger S. J. (1974) Pericardiocentesis. *Vet. Clin. N. Am.* **4**(2), 403.

Ettinger S. J. and Suter P. F. (1970) *Canine Cardiology.* Philadelphia, Saunders.

Eyster G. E. and Evans A. T. (1974) Open-heart surgery in the dog. In: Kirk R. W. (ed.), *Current Veterinary Therapy V.* Philadelphia, Saunders.

Eyster G. E., Eyster J. T., Cords G. B. et al. (1976) Patent ductus arteriosus in the dog: characteristics of occurrence and results of surgery in one hundred consecutive cases. *J. Am. Vet. Med. Assoc.* **168,** 435.

Eyster G. E., Weber W., Chi S. et al. (1976) Mitral valve prosthesis for correction of mitral regurgitation in a dog. *J. Am. Vet. Med. Assoc.* **168,** 1115.

Hamlin R. L. (1977) New ideas in the management of heart failure in dogs. *J. Am. Vet. Med. Assoc.* **171,** 114.

Hamlin R. L. and Kittleson M. D. (1982) Clinical experience with hydralazine for treatment of otherwise intractable cough in dogs and apparent left-sided heart failure. *J. Am. Vet. Med. Assoc.* **180,** 1327.

Hamlin R. L., Pipers F. S., Carter H. L. et al. (1973) Treatment of heart failure in dogs without use of digitalis glycosides. *Vet. Med. (S.A.C.)* **68,** 349.

Herrtage M. E., Hall L. W. and English T. A. H. (1983) Surgical correction of the tetralogy of Fallot in a dog. *J. Small Anim. Pract.* **24,** 51.

Kittleson M. D., Eyster G. E., Knowlen G. G., Olivier N. B. and Anderson L. K. (1985) Efficacy of digoxin administration in dogs with idiopathic congestive cardiomyopathy. *J. Am. Vet. Med. Assoc.* **186,** 162.

Kittleson M. D., Eyster G. E., Olivier N. B. and Anderson L. K. (1983) Oral hydralazine therapy for chronic mitral regurgitation in the dog. *J. Am. Vet. Med. Assoc.* **182,** 125.

Kittleson M. D. and Hamlin R. L. (1983) Hydralazine pharmacodynamics in the dog. *Am. J. Vet. Res.* **44,** 1501.

McIntosh J. J. (1981) The use of vasodilators in treatment of congestive heart failure: a review. *J. Am. Anim. Hosp. Assoc.* **17,** 225.

Thomas W. P. (1980) Long-term therapy of chronic congestive heart failure in the dog and cat. In: Kirk R. W. (ed.), *Current Veterinary Therapy VII.* Philadelphia, Saunders.

Chapter 15

Cardiac Arrest and Resuscitation

A maximum of 4 minutes is available before brain damage occurs.
Usually represents ventricular standstill/fibrillation—*dysrhythmias.*
   Predisposition for these dysrhythmias is created by:
1. Hypoxia.
2. Acidosis.
3. Excess catecholamine (sympathetic) activity:
   excitement, surgical manipulation, shock.
4. Toxaemias—uraemia, hepatic failure, electrolyte disturbances.
5. Hypothermia.
6. Excess of certain anaesthetic agents (e.g. halothane).
7. Hypotension or hypovolaemia.

Signs and findings

   a. Collapse.
   b. Respirations: cessation or rapid and shallow.
   c. Pallor or cyanosis, slow capillary refill.
   d. Loss of pulse and audible heart sounds.
   e. Dilated, unresponsive pupils.

Differential diagnosis

Seizure/syncope/airway obstruction or respiratory arrest.

Routine for resuscitation

   a. Give a single very strong thrust to the left ventral thorax.
   b. Establish an airway:

  i. Introduce a cuffed endotracheal tube.
  ii. Lower the head to drain any secretions.
  iii. Use suction (with a syringe and polythene tube if necessary).
  c. Stop anaesthetic gases and ventilate the lungs:
  i. With oxygen if available (20–30 times/min).
  ii. By blowing down the tube if necessary (10–20 times/min).
  d. Use external cardiac massage.
  Compress the thorax laterally about 60 times/min—in a ventro-dorsal direction with one hand below (best with narrow thorax).

N.B.

  i. Stop to allow inflation of the lungs every 5–10 sec.
  ii. Check for spontaneous respirations and heart beat and pupillary light reflex.
  iii. Check pupils.
  iv. Monitor the pulse.
  e. If still no heart beat after 2 minutes:
  i. Inject 1–5 ml calcium chloride (dilute to 5 per cent) i.v. or into the left ventricle.
  ii. Give 1–10 ml (of 8·4 per cent) sodium bicarbonate intravenously.
  f. If an ECG is available, check the dysrhythmia:
  i. If *ventricular standstill*:
  Inject 0·2–1·0 ml of adrenaline (1 : 10000)
  or 0·5–1·0 ml of isoprenaline (1 : 500) (Suscardia; Pharmax) into the left ventricle.
  ii. If *ventricular fibrillation*:
  Inject 0·5–5·0 ml lignocaine (2 per cent) (Xylocard; Astra)—into the left ventricle.
  Inject 0·2–1·0 ml of adrenaline (: 10000)
  —into the left ventricle.
  (Defibrillate with DC shock if available.)
  Repeat *c* and *d* again.
  g. If no heart beat is detected after 2–3 minutes, employ internal massage:
  i. Open the thoracic cavity rapidly.
  ii. Squeeze the heart from apex to base (60/min).
  Observe strong activity for 5–10 min, then close the chest.
  h. Set up an intravenous drip if the heart has responded:
  i. Isotonic saline, with
  ii. Sodium bicarbonate (5–20 ml of 8·4 per cent).
  iii. Introduce isoprenaline at 1 mg/200 ml of the drip.
  Monitor central venous pressure if possible
  (keep below 10 cm of water)

    i. Warm the patient and continue to monitor closely—ECG?

    j. Further therapy:
Dopamine (Intropin; Arnar-Stone) 40 mg in 500 ml of drip—if the pulse is still weak.

N.B.

    a. A resuscitation box containing these drugs and instructions is valuable (Lucke and Waterman, 1977).

    b. Fairly simple modern monitors (audible/visual) are now available for use during anaesthesia.

    c. Other dysrhythmias often precede arrest.

    d. ECG may show normal activity for minutes after effective stroke volume has failed and the presence of a normal rhythm does not guarantee recovery.

REFERENCES AND FURTHER READING

Breznock E. M. and Kagan K. G. (1978) Chemical cardioversion of electrically-induced ventricular fibrillation in dogs. *Am. J. Vet. Res.* **39,** 971.

Clark D. R. (1977) Recognition and treatment of cardiac emergencies. *J. Am. Vet. Med. Assoc.* **171,** 98.

Lucke J. N. and Waterman A. (1977) A portable resuscitation box for use in anaesthetic emergencies. *J. Small Anim. Pract.* **18,** 423.

Chapter 16

Oesophageal Disorders

1. Cricopharyngeal achalasia (congenital/acquired).
2. Pharyngeal inco-ordination? (especially Irish Setters).
3. Megaloesophagus (dilation)
   (Congenital/acquired, especially Irish Setters, German Shepherds); occasionally associated with myasthenia gravis, neuropathies.
4. Vascular ring stricture (especially persistent right aortic arch).
5. Oesophageal diverticulum (developmental or acquired).
6. Oesophageal foreign body, especially bones
   (especially Scottish type terriers) also needles, fish-hooks, sticks.
7. Oesophagitis:
   a. Reflux—under anaesthesia? (Pearson et al., 1978)
      —with hiatus hernia (uncommon).
   b. Ingestion of corrosives (e.g. paraquat, phenolics).
   May develop into *stricture.*
8. Neoplasia (rare).
9. *(Spirocerca lupi: rare).*
10. Extrinsic pressure (neoplasia).

Signs

   a. Oesophageal disorders usually cause *regurgitation* of undigested material ± mucus shortly after ingestion.
      But food (+ saliva) may be brought back some hours later.
   b. Often excess salivation and failure to swallow saliva.
   c. There may also be dysphagia, aerophagia, coughing.
   d. Usually not much loss of appetite (except 6, 7, *above*).
   e. Failure to swallow food (especially 1, 2, *above*).

Findings

- *a.* May be able to feel a flaccid oesophagus (3, 4, *above*).
- *b.* May hear material in the oesophagus (3, 4, *above*).
- *c.* There may be inhalation pneumonia following regurgitation.
- *d.* Oesophageal perforation and fistula (*see* p. 16) causing dyspnoea and pyrexia, can occur with (6, *above*).

Investigations

- *a.* Give a test meal to check the dog's behaviour.
- *b.* Endoscopy is very helpful, under general anaesthesia (p. 117).
- *c.* Radiology: plain films (air/food in dilated oesophagus) and films following a barium swallow (p. 118) are very important.

General management

- *a.* Liquidize food (though dried foods may help).
- *b.* Feed frequently.
- *c.* Feed from a height, with the dog standing on hind legs.

Specific treatments

- *a.* Cricopharyngeal achalasia, vascular ring structure, oesophageal stricture or hiatus hernia may require surgical correction.
- *b.* Megaloesophagus: no effective treatment (management may help).
- *c.* Oesophagitis:
  - i. Aluminium hydroxide orally (e.g. Mucaine; Wyeth).
  - ii. Metoclopramide (Emequell; Beecham) 0·5 mg/kg b.d.
  - iii. Cimetidine (Tagamet; SK & F) tablets.
- *d.* Oesophageal foreign body:
  - i. *Gently* push into stomach (with stomach tube?).
  - ii. Gently remove with alligator forceps under general anaesthetic and after giving a muscle relaxant? Via an endoscope. With fluoroscopic screening, if available.
  - iii. Oesophagotomy is necessary if any evidence of penetration is noted (Ryan and Greene, 1975).

N.B. Oesophageal perforation or stricture is a serious complication of oesophageal foreign bodies or oesophageal ulceration.

REFERENCES AND FURTHER READING

Harvey C. E., O'Brien J. A., Durie V. R. et al. (1974) Megaesophagus in the dog: a clinical survey of 79 cases. *J. Am. Vet. Med. Assoc.* **165**, 262.

Holmberg D. L. and Presnell P. L. (1979) Vascular ring anomalies: case report and brief review. *Canad. Vet. J.* **20**, 78.

Houlton J. E. F., Herrtage M. E., Taylor P. M. and Watkins S. B. (1985) Thoracic oesophageal foreign bodies in the dog: a review of ninety cases. *J. Small Anim. Pract.* **26**, 521.

Lawson D. D. and Pirie H. M. (1966) Conditions of the canine oesophagus. II Vascular rings, achalasia and perioesophageal lesions. *J. Small. Anim. Pract.* **7**, 117.

Pearson H. (1966) Conditions of the canine oesophagus. I Foreign bodies in the oesophagus. *J. Small Anim. Pract.* **7**, 107.

Pearson H., Darke P. G. G., Kelly D. F. et al. (1978) Reflux oesophagitis and stricture formation after anaesthesia: a review of seven cases in dogs and cats. *J. Small Anim. Pract.* **19**, 341.

Rawlings C. A., Dhein C. R. M., Rosin E. et al. (1980) Esophageal hiatal hernia and eventration of the diaphragm with resultant gastroesophageal reflux. *J. Am. Anim. Hosp. Assoc.* **16**, 517.

Ryan W. W. and Greene R. W. (1975) The conservative management of esophageal foreign bodies and their complications: a review of 66 cases in dogs and cats. *J. Am. Anim. Hosp. Assoc.* **11**, 243.

Watrous B. J. (1983) Esophageal disease. In: Ettinger S. J. (ed.), *Textbook of Veterinary Internal Medicine,* 2nd Ed. Philadelphia, Saunders.

Chapter 17

Gastric Disorders

A. ACUTE GASTRIC DISORDERS

1. Gastritis—very common—due to:
   - *a.* Ingestion of irritants:
       - i. Decaying materials.
       - ii. Toxins (lead, fertilizers).
       - iii. Drugs (glycosides, salicylates).
       - iv. Mechanical (bones/grass?).
       - v. Skin medications.
   - *b.* Infections:
       - i. Distemper, parvovirus, hepatitis, coronavirus.
       - ii. Leptospirosis (other bacteria?).
       - iii. Ascarids (mainly intestinal irritation).
   - *c.* Toxaemias: uraemia, pyometra.
   - *d.* Allergy?

   Very commonly also associated with enteritis.
2. Gastric dilatation/torsion:
   - *a.* Dilatation—may occur in any breed.
   - *b.* Torsion—tends to follow in deep-chested breeds.

   Aetiology:
       - i. Aerophagia, vagal inhibition (stress) (Caywood et al., 1976).
       - ii. Pyloric or duodenal obstruction? Gastric dysrhythmia?
       - iii. (Rapid fermentation of ingesta?) (especially cereals?)
3. Pyloric obstruction (polyp/foreign body/stenosis).
4. Haemorrhagic syndrome ('Haemorrhagic gastroenteritis'—HGE).
   Aetiology uncertain—probably endotoxic shock (Burrows, 1977).
5. Overeating (especially puppies).

Signs

    a. True vomiting—may be unproductive.
    b. Depression, anorexia, abdominal discomfort.
    c. Thirst—may vomit water back.
    d. Haematemesis (especially 1*c,* 3 and 4 *above*)?

Findings

    a. Anterior abdominal pain.
    b. Bloat and shock (2 *above*).
    c. Rapidly-developing dehydration.

Initial management

Simple gastritis is usually self-limiting:
    a. Starve totally of food (and milk) for 24 hours.
    b. Offer small quantities of water frequently (if retained).
    c. Administer gastric sedative,
        e.g. aluminium hydroxide (Aludrox or Mucaine; Wyeth).
    d. Offer bland food next day
        (carbohydrate, boiled fish or chicken and rice).
If vomiting persists, or shock or dehydration develop, follow the
procedure for acute abdominal disorders (Chapter 20).

Specific treatment

    a. Foreign bodies and pyloric obstruction should be relieved
        surgically.
    b. For gastric dilatation/torsion (Walshaw and Johnston, 1976):
        i. Introduce an intravenous drip (0·9 per cent saline: 50 ml/
           kg body weight in first hour with 5 ml (5 mEq)/kg body
           weight bicarbonate. Check and correct acid-base if
           possible.
        ii. Administer glucocorticoids and antibiotics at a high
           dose.
        iii. Introduce a lubricated stomach tube (foal size—9·5 mm) to
           try gently to deflate the stomach.
           If necessary: lift dog by forelimbs and rotate body axis. If
           unsuccessful: gently release gas through a needle (18
           gauge) then try a stomach tube again.
        iv. Wash out stomach with warm saline and drain.
        v. Assess and treat any cardiac dysrhythmia
           (Chapter 11).

vi. Consider gastrostomy under local anaesthetic in the right paracostal region—closed after 12 hours (Parks and Greene, 1976).

vii. When the circulation is restored: check position of stomach by X-ray. (Funkquist, 1979).

If gastric torsion: laporotomy and gastropexy may be necessary.

B. CHRONIC GASTRIC DISORDERS

1. Gastritis:
   a. Commonly due to *toxaemias* (e.g. uraemia or hepatic failure).
   b. (Rarely—a specific disorder—chronic gastritis [Huxtable and Mills, 1978] or hypertrophic gastritis [Van Kruiningen, 1977].
2. Neoplasia:
   a. Adenocarcinoma (especially ageing Scottish-type terriers).
   b. Benign polyps (especially pylorus).
   c. Other sarcomata.
3. Ulceration:
   Association with hepatic disease and with mastocytomas;
   also occurs late in chronic renal failure (uraemia).
4. Pyloric dysfunction;
   a. Congenital hypertrophy or stenosis (especially young Boxers).
   b. Acquired stenosis or spasm.
5. Foreign body:
   either
   a. Incidental finding, causing little disturbance (bone, gravel).
   or
   b. Causing intermittent pyloric obstruction (e.g. a ball).

Signs

Often vague and variable:
   a. True vomiting:
      i. May be intermittent.
      ii. Variable time after feeding.
      iii. May be haematemesis (with 1, 2a, 3, 5, *above*).
   b. Weight loss.
   c. Appetite variable—may be depressed   } (especially 1, 2, 3
   d. Depression, abdominal pain.   }   *above*)
   e. May be melaena (2a, 3, *above*).
   f. Thirst may be increased.

Findings

  a. Anterior abdominal pain.
  b. Lesions are rarely palpable.
  c. Anaemia (1*a*, 2*a*, 3, *above*).

Investigations

  a. Radiology and a barium meal (Chapter 35):
      But radiographs may need careful interpretation (especially 2*a*, 3, *above*).
  b. Endoscopy (especially 2, 3, *above*) (*see* Chapter 19).
  c. Exploratory laparotomy and biopsy if necessary.

Specific treatment

  a. Neoplasms can be sometimes removed (not 2*c*, *above*) but adenocarcinoma may require extensive surgery.
  b. Gastrotomy for a foreign body.
  c. Pyloromyotomy (Ramstedt's operation) for (4 *above*).
  d. Peptic ulceration and chronic gastritis:
      i. Surgical excision of ulcerated mucosa?
      ii. Frequent feeding of small quantities of bland food.
      iii. Drugs: magnesium hydroxide (Milk of Magnesia); aluminium hydroxide (mucaine; Wyeth); cimetidine (Tagamet; Smith, Kline & French) 20–100 mg orally t.d.s.
  N.B. Must avoid: salicylates; anticholinergics; corticosteroids.

REFERENCES AND FURTHER READING

Anderson N. V. (1980) *Veterinary Gastroenterology.* Philadelphia, Lea & Febiger.
Burrows C. F. (1977) Canine hemorrhagic gastroenteritis. *J. Am. Anim. Hosp. Assoc.* **13**, 451.
Caywood D., Teague H. D., Jackson D. A. et al. (1976) Gastric gas analysis in the canine gastric dilatation—volvulus syndrome. *J. Am. Anim. Hosp. Assoc.* **12**, 173.
Funkquist B. (1979) Gastric torsion in the dog—I. Radiological picture during non-surgical treatment related to pathological anatomy and to the further clinical course. *J. Small Anim. Pract.* **20**, 73.
Gaskell C. J., Gibbs C. and Pearson H. (1974) Sliding hiatus hernia with reflex oesophagitis in two dogs. *J. Small Anim. Pract.* **15**, 503.
Happé R. P. van der Gaag I. and Wolvekamp W. Th. C. (1981) Pyloric stenosis caused by hypertrophic gastritis in three dogs. *J. Small Anim. Pract.* **22**, 7.
Huxtable C. F. and Mills J. N. (1982) Chronic hypertrophic gastritis in a dog: successful treatment by partial gastrectomy. *J. Small Anim. Pract.* **23**, 639.
Murray M., Robinson P. B., McKeating F. J. et al. (1972) Peptic ulceration in the dog: A clinico-pathological study. *Vet. Rec.* **91**, 441.

Murray M., Robinson P. B., McKeating F. J. et al. (1972) Primary gastric neoplasia in the dog: a clinico-pathological study. *Vet. Rec.* **91,** 474.

Parks J. L. and Greene R. W. (1976) Tube gastrostomy for the treatment of gastric volvulus. *J. Am. Anim. Hosp. Assoc.* **12,** 168.

Pass M. A. and Johnston D. E. (1973) Treatment of gastric dilation and torsion in the dog. Gastric decompression by gastrotomy under local analgesia. *J. Small Anim. Pract.* **14,** 131.

Twedt D. C. and Wingfield W. E. (1983) Diseases of the stomach. In: Ettinger S. J. (ed.), *Textbook of Veterinary Internal Medicine,* 2nd Ed. Philadelphia, Saunders.

Van Kruiningen H. J. (1977) Giant hypertrophic gastritis of Basenji dogs. *Vet. Path.* **14,** 19.

Walshaw R. and Johnston D. E. (1976) Treatment of gastric dilatation-volvulus by gastric decompression and patient stabilization before major surgery. *J. Am. Anim. Hosp. Assoc.* **12,** 162.

Chapter 18

Differential Diagnosis of Vomiting

It is important to differentiate true vomiting from regurgitation or retching, as the approach to investigation and management is dissimilar.

DEFINITIONS

1. True vomiting (usually *gastric*)

A complex mechanism activated by the medullary centre.
- *a.* Nasopharynx and larynx close:
- *b.* Gastric fundus and oesophagus relax (gastric stasis and atony).
- *c.* Pylorus and abdominal and respiratory muscles contract
  → forceful expulsion of stomach contents
  —may also be duodenal-gastric reflux.

Associated signs

Apprehension, restlessness, distress, lip licking, swallowing movements. Salivation, retching with head lowered and breath held. Abdominal muscles in rhythmic contractions.

Character of vomitus

- *a.* Typically: mucus, froth, food (variably digested).
- *b.* Commonly: bile (duodenal reflux).
- *c.* Occasionally:
  - i. Blood (dark brown if long in the stomach) (ulcer, neoplasm, foreign body, haemorrhagic gastroenteritis).
  - ii. 'Faeces' (intestinal obstruction) (dark brown contents are probably *not* faeces).

VOMITING

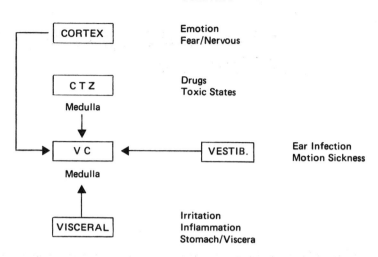

Fig. 7. Summary of the stimuli for vomiting. CTZ, chemoreceptor trigger zone; VC, vomiting centre.

    d. pH is usually < 4 if of gastric origin only; 4–7 if bile is present (duodenal reflux).
    e. Vomiting of solids rather than liquids suggests *partial obstruction.*

Relationship to feeding
    a. Variable in gastric disorders—may be ½–6 hours later.
    b. Often thirsty—then vomit water back.
    c. *Rarely* projectile vomiting in dogs.

Stimuli for true vomiting (at the vomiting centre, *Fig.* 7)
    a. Visceral irritation/stretching/pain
    (reflex receptors between pharynx and rectum
       → vomiting centre via autonomic nerves):
      i. Irritation or inflammation of alimentary tract.
     ii. Inflammation of abdominal viscera including the peritoneum (hepatitis, pancreatitis, peritonitis).
    iii. Distension/pressure on or in viscera:
        Gastric overload or dilatation.
        Abdominal neoplasia.
        Gastro-intestinal obstruction.

   b. CNS irritation or stimulation of the chemoreceptor trigger zone (CTZ):(chemoreceptors trigger the vomiting centre):
      i. Toxaemia (uraemia, pyometra, hepatic failure).
      ii. Iatrogenic (salicylates, glycosides, opiates).
   c. Other CNS stimulation:
      i. Motion (travel sickness or vestibular lesions?).
      ii. Emotion (fear, excitement, attention-seeking).
      iii. Psychological or epilepsy.
      iv. Odours/tastes/pain
   d. CNS lesions (encephalitis or meningitis).

2. Regurgitation (usually oesophageal)

Usually very soon after ingestion.

Few prodromal signs
   a. No retching or abdominal contraction.
   b. Abrupt, brief, not very distressing.
   c. Mouth open, mandible fixed, little effort (passive).

Associated signs
   a. Coughing, salivation are common.
   b. May re-eat food unless a *painful* disorder.
   c. May be aerophagia, gulping, swallowing.
   d. May be discomfort in swallowing.

Character of vomitus
   a. Undigested *bolus* or tube of recognisable food or saliva.
   b. pH > 6. No bile.

3. Pharyngeal retching

Signs
   a. Distress in attempts to swallow.
   b. Food hooked back with the tongue.
      → *immediate* return of unswallowed food.
   c. May pass down the nose—especially liquids.
   d. May be coughing as the animal swallows liquid.
   e. Retraction of the lips, tongue movements.
   f. Head bobbing during attempts to swallow.

4. Other retching (especially toxaemias, paroxysmal coughing)
   a. Ineffectual and involuntary attempts at vomiting.
   b. Unproductive abdominal effort with the head lowered.
   c. May follow paroxysms of unproductive coughing (Chapter 5).

DIFFERENTIAL DIAGNOSIS OF VOMITING, REGURGITATION, RETCHING AND DYSPHAGIA

1. Acute vomiting

  a. Gastritis, gastric dilatation.
  b. Intestinal obstruction: foreign body, tumour, stricture, intussusception, volvulus, strangulated hernia, ileus.
  c. Pyloric obstruction (foreign body, polyp).
  d. Acute haemorrhagic syndrome (HGE).
  e. Over-eating.
  f. Motion sickness.
  g. Toxins/poisons/drugs.
  h. Systemic infections (Distemper, hepatitis, parvovirus).
  i. Other acute abdominal disorders (Chapter 20).

2. Recurrent/chronic vomiting

  a. Scavenging and recurrent gastritis.
  b. Toxaemias: uraemia; pyometra; hepatic failure; diabetes mellitus; hypoadrenocorticalism.
  c. Pressure on GI tract: hepatic/pancreatic/splenic tumours.
  d. Visceral inflammation: peritonitis; pancreatitis; hepatitis; nephritis.
  e. Variable pyloric obstruction: neoplasia; stenosis; spasm; foreign body.
  f. Gastric ulceration or neoplasia.
  g. Psychological/behavioural vomiting or CNS disease.
  h. Incomplete obstruction: intestinal foreign body; tumour; stricture/adhesion; intussusception.
  i. Chronic pancreatitis.
  j. Gastritis chronica or hyperacidity?
  k. Hypertrophic gastritis.

3. Regurgitation/retching

  a. Megaloesophagus.
  b. Pharyngitis or tonsillitis.
  c. Cricopharyngeal achalasia.
  d. Vascular ring stricture.
  e. Pharyngeal incoordination.
  f. Oesophageal foreign body.
  g. Oesophagitis/oesophageal stricture.
  h. Oesophageal diverticulum.
  i. Hiatus hernia
  j. Gastro-oesophageal intussusception.

   k. Peri-oesophageal masses: abscesses, lymphomegaly, neoplasms.
   l. (Oesophageal neoplasia).
  m. Following coughing (*see* Chapter 5).

4. Dysphagia

(Difficulty or pain in swallowing, while maintaining a desire to eat.) May
be hesitation in swallowing or repeated gagging. Usually extension and
lowering of the head and neck during swallowing:

   a. Mouth
       i. Stomatitis/glossitis
        (caustic, immune-mediated, viral, vitamin B deficiency).
      ii. Tumour.
     iii. Foreign body.
     iv. Mandible fracture or luxation.
      v. Craniomandibular osteopathy.
     vi. Temporal muscles: eosinophilic myositis/atrophy.
    vii. Trigeminal paralysis.
   viii. Osteoporosis ('rubber jaw').
   b. Pharynx
       i. Pharyngitis.
      ii. Tonsillitis.
     iii. Tonsil tumour.
     iv. Foreign body.
   c. External oesophageal obstruction
       i. Neck tumours (thyroid, abscesses).
      ii. Mediastinal tumours (thymic, cardiac).
     iii. Lung tumour.
     iv. Vascular ring stricture.
   d. Oesophageal disease
       i. Cricopharyngeal achalasia.
      ii. Megaloesophagus.
     iii. Oesophagitis/stricture.
     iv. Oesophageal foreign body.
      v. Oesophageal diverticulum.
   e. Other disorders
       i. Myasthenia gravis.
      ii. Rabies.
     iii. Tetanus.
     iv. Botulism.

MANAGEMENT OF VOMITING

   a. Treat any cause (including withdrawal of any drugs).
   b. Block the CTZ? (dopamine antagonists):

      i. Acetylpromazine, chlorpromazine.

      ii. Metoclopramide (also prevents gastric stasis).

   c. Block the vomiting centre?

      i. Acetylpromazine.

      ii. Fentanyl.

   d. Behavioural disorders—megestrol?

FURTHER READING

Anderson N. V. (1980) *Veterinary Gastroenterology.* Philadelphia, Lea & Febiger.

Pearson H. (1970) The differential diagnosis of persistent vomiting in the young dog. *J. Small Anim. Pract.* **11**, 403.

Yoxall A. T. (1980) The vomiting dog. In: Yoxall A. T. and Hird J. F. R. (ed.), *Physiological Basis of Small Animal Medicine.* Oxford, Blackwell Scientific Publications.

Chapter 19

Investigation of Persistent Vomiting/Regurgitation

Persistent vomiting may indicate serious disease, or it may be only behavioural. Detailed investigation is required to diagnose some gastric disorders.

History

Note carefully:

    a. Age and general health:
        i. Congenital disorder?
        ii. Neoplasia?
        iii. Other systemic disease? (uraemia, pyometra).
        iv. Weight loss.
        v. Previous health.
    b. Animal's precise behaviour at the time of vomiting:
        i. True vomit or regurgitation (Chapter 18)?
        ii. Cough and retching rather than vomit?
        iii. Salivation, re-eating?
    c. Frequency of occurrence.
    d. Timing in relation to feeding (upper or lower tract?).
    e. Presence or absence of diarrhoea, nature of faeces.
    f. Appetite and diet (access to rubbish/irritants/foreign body?).
    g. Can the dog eat normally?
    h. Character of vomitus:
        i. Froth/mucus/blood/bile?
        ii. Solids *and* liquids vomited?
    i. Any coughing? (inhalation of regurgitated material?)

    j. Breed susceptibility:
        i. Irish Setter, German Shepherd (megaloesophagus).
        ii. Boxer (pyloric stenosis).
        iii. Scottish type terriers (oesophageal foreign body).

Examination

    a. Signs of debilitation and other systemic disease?
    b. Palpation of the pharynx and neck
        (Oesophageal dilatation?)
        (Masses pressing on the oesophagus?)
    c. Abdominal palpation:
        i. Stomach is poorly palpable—but there may be *pain.*
        ii. Intestinal lesions or foreign body palpable?
        iii. Abdominal masses palpable?
    d. Thorax
        i. Muffling of sounds? (mass).
        ii. Fluid in the oesophagus? (megaloesophagus).

Further investigations

    a. Examination of vomitus—pH, bile, blood (Chapter 18)?
    b. Check blood and urine samples for evidence of *toxaemia*
        (plasma urea, liver enzymes).
    c. Test meal—to observe the pattern of vomiting or
        regurgitation.
    d. *Endoscopy*—a valuable procedure (Heppe and Van der Gaag,
        1983).
        A flexible fibreoptic endoscope is preferable to a rigid tube for
        examining the *pylorus* (for tumours, ulcers, foreign body).
        Procedure:
        i. General anaesthesia and tracheal intubation.
        ii. Dog in lateral recumbency.
        iii. Extend the neck and draw the tongue forwards.
        iv. Insert a mouth gag to protect the endoscope.
        v. Pass the lubricated endoscope *gently* down the
           oesophagus—manipulate around obstructions
           (thoracic inlet/over the heart), and introduce *gently*
           into the stomach.
        vi. May have to remove saliva (suction?).
        vii. Must manipulate the flexible endoscope around the
           stomach to observe the pylorus—may also need to
           manipulate the dog.
        viii. Best view of the oesophagus is often obtained on
           withdrawal of the endoscope.

    ix. May be able to biopsy a lesion with forceps.

    x. May be able to remove a foreign body with forceps or a snare.

Potential findings:

    i. Oesophagus:

        Foreign bodies.

        Megaloesophagus.

        Oesophagitis (ulceration).

        Strictures.

        Diverticula.

        Neoplasia.

    ii. Stomach:

        Foreign bodies.

        Ulceration.

        Neoplasia.

  e. Upper alimentary radiology.

An important procedure (*see also* Chapter 35):

    i. The animal should be starved for 24 hours.

    ii. Oesophageal function is affected by anaesthesia and sedation—avoid if possible.

    iii. Must examine *plain films* first.

    iv. *Two* views (lateral and ventrodorsal) of the thorax and/or the anterior abdomen are essential.

    v. Contrast radiology (usually with barium):

        Food and barium (Micropaque; Nicholas Lab.) mixed—for the oesophagus.

        Liquid Micropaque 5–10 ml —for suspected gastric foreign body.

        Liquid Micropaque 5 ml/kg for other gastric lesions.

Take immediate, 10 minute, ½, 2, 4 and 6 hour films to assess gastric emptying and persistence of 'lesions'.

Double contrast (with air by stomach tube) may give a good image for the detection of gastric lesions.

Iodine solutions (e.g. Gastrografin; Schering) should be used if there is any sign of oesophageal penetration.

Information sought

  a. Position of oesophagus and stomach.

  b. Patency of oesophagus and pylorus.

  c. Presence and site of lesions within and outwith the tract.

  d. Speed of emptying of the stomach:

    i. Normally   { starts 5–30 min.   complete in 3–5 hours.

    ii. Delayed by pyloric lesions or spasm.

N.B. Indentations on gastric films may merely represent rugae or peristalsis; check for *persistence* of apparent lesions.

Potential findings

   a. Oesophagus
      i. Foreign body.
      ii. Megaloesophagus.
      iii. Vascular ring strictures.
      iv. Diverticulum.
      v. Stricture.
      vi. Hiatus hernia.
   b. Stomach:
      i. Foreign body.
      ii. Neoplasia.
      iii. (Ulceration?)
      iv. Dilatation.
      v. Pyloric stenosis.

Fluoroscopy (image intensification) is potentially very helpful following a barium meal for gastric lesions.

If a lesion is located, then exploratory laparotomy and, if necessary, gastrotomy and biopsy are indicated.

However, exploratory surgery is *not* an adequate substitute for thorough clinical investigation.

General notes

   a. Occasional vomiting is not uncommon in normal dogs, e.g. with:
      i. Recurrent scavenging
      ii. Psychogenic causes.
      iii. Nursing bitches.
   Always assess and reassess whether:
      i. Signs of debility or toxaemia are present
         (depression, weight loss, anorexia)
      ii. Further developments have occurred—reinvestigate?
         e.g. gastric neoplasia may be very slow in developing, and radiographic findings may be uncertain at the time of first examination.
   b. Persistent vomiting is very tiring and may cause irreversible electrolyte changes, with hypovolaemia—therefore intravenous fluid therapy is *very important* until a diagnosis and cure is established.
   c. Inhalation pneumonia may result from recurrent or severe vomiting or regurgitation, especially if the dog is weak or debilitated.

REFERENCES AND FURTHER READING

Anderson N. V. (1980) *Veterinary Gastroenterology.* Philadelphia, Lea & Febiger.

Happe R. P. and Van der Gaag I. (1983) Endoscopic examination of esophagus, stomach and duodenum in the dog. *J. Am. Anim. Hosp. Assoc.* **19,** 197.

Johnson G. F. (1980) Gastroscopy. In: Anderson N. V. (ed.), *Veterinary Gastroenterology.* Philadelphia, Lea & Febiger.

Kleine L. J. (1974) Radiographic examination of the esophagus in dogs and cats. *Vet. Clin. N. Am.* **4,** 663.

O'Brien T. R. (1978) *Radiographic Diagnosis of Abdominal Disorders in the Dog and Cat.* Philadelphia, Saunders.

O'Brien J. A. (1980) Esophagoscopy. In: Anderson N. V. (ed.) *Veterinary Gastroenterology.* Philadelphia. Lea & Febiger.

Sullivan M. and Miller A. (1985) Endoscopy (fibreoptic) of the oesophagus and stomach in the dog with persistent regurgitation or vomiting. *J. Small Anim. Pract.* **26,** 369.

Chapter 20

Acute Abdominal Disorders

Most cases of acute vomiting (e.g. due to gastritis) cease within a few hours. Persistent acute and severe vomiting is serious, as fluid, electrolyte and acid—base disturbances occur, and shock develops.

The term 'acute abdomen' is used in man, and it can equally be applied to disorders causing acute and severe vomiting, often with abdominal pain and with the rapid development of shock, in dogs. The correct management of these cases is critically important.

Typical signs

- *a.* Vomiting and retching.
- *b.* Abdominal pain.
- *c.* Depression, anorexia.
- *d.* Dehydration, shock and hypothermia.
- *e.* May also be diarrhoea, pyrexia.

The syndrome may be caused by a number of life-threatening disorders not readily differentiated by simple clinical examination.

Potential differential diagnoses

- *a.* Gastrointestinal tract irritation:
  - Gastroenteritis.
- *b.* Intestinal obstruction:
  - i. Stricture.
  - ii. Foreign body.
  - iii. Intussusception.
  - iv. Volvulus.

      v. Strangulated hernia.
     vi. Paralytic ileus.
    vii. Neoplasms (when advanced).
  c. Acute disorders of intra-abdominal organs:
      i. Hepatitis.
     ii. Pancreatitis.
    iii. Nephritis.
    iv. Peritonitis.
     v. Prostatitis.
    vi. Splenic torsion.
   vii. Torsion of a retained testicle.
  viii. Urinary obstruction.
    ix. (Metritis?)
  d. Miscellaneous:
      i. Hypoadrenocorticalism (Addisonian crisis).
     ii. Gastric dilatation.
    iii. Ruptured ulcer or neoplasm in the alimentary tract.
    iv. Poisoning (heavy metal, organophosphates).

Fortunately, with careful fluid therapy and management a number of these disorders are reversible. Treatment may be approached in a similar fashion, even if the precise cause is uncertain.

Suggested management approach

  a. Examine the dog rapidly but carefully.
    Check:
      i. History:
        Access to foreign body, poisons.
        Possibility of trauma.
        Pattern of vomiting, defaecation, urination.
     ii. Palpation—site of pain:
        Renal/gastric/hepatic/intestinal/prostatic?
    iii. Peristalsis (auscultate?):
        Increase = gastritis.
        Decrease = peritonitis; obstruction; toxaemia?
    iv. Other signs of toxaemia?
  b. Palpate and X-ray for signs of intestinal or urinary obstruction (foreign body, intussusception, urinary calculi, ruptured bladder). If present: prepare for surgery.
  c. Use abdominal paracentesis if there is any sign of effusion.
  d. Take blood samples for:
    Routine haematology
    Urea, amylase, liver enzyme levels.
    Glucose.

Take urine for analysis (by catheter—with care):
Concentration—high: hypovolaemia?
low: renal failure?

e. Introduce intravenous fluid therapy e.g. 40 ml/kg body weight of Hartmann's solution in 1 hour, followed by 20–40 ml/kg body weight.

f. Administer drugs:
   i. 4 mg/kg body weight pethidine i.m.
   ii. Broad-spectrum antibiotic (high dose).
   iii. Glucocorticoids:
        Dexamethasone (0·1 mg/kg body weight i.v.).
        Betamethasone (similar dose).
   iv. Spasmolytics:
        Atropine (0·3–1 mg s.c.).
        Hyoscine (Buscopan; Boehringer) 5–10 mg i.m.
        Menthidizate (Isaverin; Bayer) 1–5 ml i.m.
   v. Central antiemetic:
        Metoclopramide (Emequell; Beecham)
        0·5–1·0 mg/kg i.v. or i.m. (*contraindicated* if foreign body obstruction).

g. Provide support:
   i. Starve for 24 hours.
   ii. Warmth.
   iii. B vitamins?
   iv. Oral gastric sedatives (e.g. Mucaine; Wyeth).
   v. Sodium bicarbonate *in the drip* 2–5 mEq/kg body weight.

h. Check urine flow within 1 hour (catheter?):
   i. If absent—reduce fluid therapy, use diuresis?
   ii. If good—maintain fluid therapy.
   Stop fluid administration if the central venous pressure is measured and it rises above 10 cm of water.

i. Surgery—if necessary
   —but only when the circulation has been restored.

Most disorders will improve with this regime, but support may be necessary for 2–3 days, by which time the results of laboratory tests may be available.

N.B.:

a. Many biochemical parameters are affected by vomiting and dehydration:
   i. Urine is usually very concentrated (oliguria).
   ii. Elevated plasma urea is expected with most of these disorders (prerenal uraemia).
   iii. Levels of glucose, amylase, liver enzymes, plasma proteins and haematology are also disturbed by most disorders.

   b. Pancreatitis:
      i. This has been treated surgically (Denny and Lucke, 1972).
      ii. If a specific diagnosis is obtained, support as above.
   c. If vomiting persists further consider:
      i. Renal failure—recheck plasma urea (Chapter 28).
      ii. Contrast radiology (barium meal).
      iii. Maintain fluid therapy.
      iv. See p. 117 for further management of persistent vomiting.

REFERENCES AND FURTHER READING

Denny H. R. and Lucke J. N. (1972) A case of acute pancreatic necrosis in the dog. *J. Small Anim. Pract.* **13,** 545.

Gibbs C. and Pearson H. (1973) The radiological diagnosis of gastrointestinal obstruction in the dog. *J. Small Anim. Pract.* **14,** 61.

Kleine L. J. (1979) Radiology of acute abdominal disorders in the dog and cat. *Comp. Cont. ed. Pract Vet.* **1,** 520 and 614.

Twedt D. C. and Grauer G. F. (1982) Fluid therapy of gastrointestinal, pancreatic and hepatic disorders. *Vet. Clin. N. Am.* **12,** 463.

Chapter 21

Disorders of the Small Intestine

The small intestine has a vast surface area, with a very rapid turnover of cells, which even comprise a portion of faeces.

Secretion and absorption of fluids takes place. The small intestine is an important barrier in immune defence, though an excess of inflammatory cells is associated with some malabsorptive disorders.

A. ACUTE INTESTINAL OBSTRUCTION

1. Complete foreign body obstruction (stones/plastic/rubber balls), especially in *young* dogs.
2. Intussusception: usually in dogs less than 1 year old, may follow acute diarrhoea/heavy ascarid infestation/neoplasia; often occurs at the ileocolic junction, but it can produce bowel prolapse.
3. Intestinal torsion (uncommon).
4. Strangulated hernia (uncommon).
5. Neoplasm or adhesion
(may cause acute obstruction, even though slowly-developing).

Signs

    a. Vomit everything—almost immediately.
    b. Depression, anorexia.
    c. Abdominal pain.
    d. Minimal faeces passed (though diarrhoea may initially be seen).
The nearer the pylorus, the more severe the signs.

125

Findings

    a. Rapid dehydration and shock.
    b. May be a palpable obstruction.
    c. Abdominal discomfort.

Investigation and management

See Chapter 20.

B. ACUTE INTESTINAL IRRITATION

1. Enteritis.
   Causes are similar to those of gastritis (Chapter 17).
   Additional agents: salmonellae, shigellae (campylobacter?).
   There is doubt as to whether bacteria are primary pathogens in dogs.
2. Haemorrhagic syndrome ('haemorrhagic gastroenteritis')
   —not a true enteritis
   —haemorrhage is associated with endotoxic shock
   (Burrows, 1977).
3. Intestinal rupture:
       a. Road accident, other abdominal trauma.
       b. Ruptured neoplasm, foreign body penetration.
         —may cause peritonitis and paralytic ileus.
4. Partial obstruction:
       a. Intussusception (especially ileocolic junction).
       b. Linear foreign body.

Signs

    a. Borborygmi.
    b. Diarrhoea±blood.
    c. Abdominal discomfort.
    d. Vomiting (variable).

Findings

    a. Abdominal discomfort.
    b. 'Gassy' feel to intestines.
    c. Shock (HGE, parvovirus, rupture?).
    d. Pyrexia (parvovirus).

Management

    a. Starve 24 hours.
    b. Oral fluids (if retained) for rehydration.

   c. Intestinal sedatives (bismuth, attapulgite, kaolin?)—some are of doubtful value.

   d. Intravenous fluid therapy if dog is dehydrated or depressed.

   e. Antibiotics only if dog is depressed, pyrexic or has dysentery.

C. CHRONIC INTESTINAL DISORDERS

1. Small intestine wall disease

   a. Lymphosarcoma (young-middle age).

   b. Villous atrophy:
      i. Idiopathic.
      ii. Viral infections.
      iii. With lymphosarcoma.

   c. Lymphangiectasia (obstruction of lymphatics) young-middle aged dogs—often a *protein-losing* disorder.

   d. Eosinophilic enteritis.
      Aetiology is uncertain (?parasitic).

   e. Other regional inflammation or infiltration (lymphocytic, plasma cell, histiocytic).

   f. Other neoplasia (especially adenocarcinoma).

2. Other digestive or absorption failures

   a. Alactasia (disaccharidase insufficiency) → milk maldigestion.

   b. 'Carrier' failures, at brush border level? (Batt, 1984). (Esp. Wheat-sensitive enteropathy in Irish setters)

3. Partial obstructions

   a. Usually—linear foreign bodies, e.g. cloth or string (needles and bones may pass through to the rectum).

   b. Partially-obstructing intussusception.

   c. Neoplasia.

4. Bacterial overgrowth

General signs of chronic intestinal disease (1–4)

   a. Diarrhoea—persistent (for investigation, *see* Chapter 23).

   b. Weight loss.

   c. Variable appetite—though sometimes increased.

   d. (Occasionally: vomiting—especially (3, *above*)).

   e. Poor skin (seborrhoea) and coat are common.

General Management

   see Page 137

5. Parasites

   a. Ascardis (Toxocara spp, Toxascaris).
   b. Tapeworms.
      i. Taenia spp.
      ii. *Echinococcus granulosus* (from hydatid cysts in herbivores).
      iii. *Dipylidium caninum* (from fleas or lice).
   c. Hookworms: *Uncinaria stenocephala (Ancylostoma caninum* is *rare* in the UK).
   d. Whipworms: *Trichuris vulpis* (mainly large intestine).
   e. Coccidia.
   f. Giardia spp.
(*c, d* and *e* may cause problems in close communities of young dogs kept in unhygienic conditions.)

Signs of parasitic infections
Often minimal, unless heavy infestations.
   a. Diarrhoea ± haemorrhage (especially *e, above*).
   b. Weight loss (not usual). Poor weight gain (esp. 5. *c. above*)
   c. Segments seen (tapeworms).
   d. Hysteria/colic/seizures in pups? (especially 5*a, above*).

Findings in parasitic infections
Minimal—may be anaemia (5*d, e, above*).
Detection requires faecal flotation, repeated if necessary.

Specific treatment for parasitic infections
   a. Ascarids:
      i. Piperazine.
      ii. Nitroscanate (Lopatol; Ciba-Geigy).
      iii. Mebendazole (Telmin KH; Crown).
      iv. Dichlorvos (Task; Tasman).
3-monthly wormings are now recommended for dogs.
   b. Tapeworms:
      i. Bunamidine (Scolaban; Wellcome).*
      ii. Praziquantel (Droncit; Bayer).
      iii. Nitroscanate (Lopatol; Ciba-Geigy).*
      iv. Mebendazole (Telmin KH; Crown). †

---

* Limited activity against Echinococcus.
† Limited activity against Dipylidium.

3-monthly dosing is recommended to eradicate Echinococcus.
- c. Other nematodes:
  - i. Dichlorvos (Task; Tasman).
  - ii. Nitroscanate (Lopatol; Ciba-Geigy).
  - iii. Mebendazole (Telmin KH; Crown).
- d. Coccidia:
  - i. Nitrofurazone
  - ii. Sulphonamides.
- e. Giardia: Metronidazole 25 mg/kg b.d. for 5 days.

6. Focal neoplasms (e.g. adenocarcinoma)

Initially no signs, then:
- a. May cause diarrhoea, weight loss.
- or b. Eventual bowel obstruction.
- or c. Bowel rupture and peritonitis.

Detected by radiography following a barium meal (Chapter 35).

7. Duodenal ulcer

Signs similar to gastric ulcer (Chapter 17), but less common (usually associated with neoplasia).

8. Paralytic ileus (or stagnant loop).

Signs

Variable—anorexia, weight loss±vomiting, diarrhoea.
Detected as an intestinal obstruction (Chapter 35).

Treatment

Resection of the affected section of intestine.

REFERENCES AND FURTHER READING

Anderson N. V. (1980) *Veterinary Gastroenterology.* Philadelphia, Lea & Febiger.

Barlough J. E. (1979) Canine giardiasis—a review. *J. Small Anim. Pract.* **20**, 613.

Batt R. M. (1980) The molecular basis of malabsorption. *J. Small Anim. Pract.* **21**, 555.

Batt R. M. (1984) Chronic small intestinal disease in the dog. *J. Small. Anim. Pract.* **25**, 707.

Bogan J. A. and Duncan J. L. (1984) Anthelmintics for dogs, cats and horses. *Br. Vet. J.* **140**, 361.

Burnie A. G., Simpson J. W., Lindsay D., and Miles R. S. (1983) The excretion of Campylobacter, Salmonellae and *Giardia lamblia* in the faeces of stray dogs. *Vet. Res. Comm.* **6**, 133.

Burrows C. F. (1977) Canine hemorrhagic gastroenteritis. *J. Am. Anim. Hosp. Assoc.* **13**, 451.

DiBartola S. P., Rogers L. S. A., Boyce J. T. and Grimm J. P. (1982) Regional enteritis in two dogs. *J. Am. Vet. Med. Assoc.* **181**, 904.

Finco D. R., Duncan J. R., Schall W. D. et al. (1973) Chronic enteric disease and hypoproteinemia in nine dogs. *J. Am. Vet. Med. Assoc.* **163**, 262.

Flesja K. and Yri T. (1977) Protein-losing enteropathy in the Lundehund. *J. Small Anim Pract.* **18**, 11.

Hayden D. W. and van Kruiningen H. J. (1973) Eosinophilic gastroenteritis in German Shepherd dogs and its relationship to visceral larva migrans. *J. Am. Vet. Med. Assoc.* **162**, 379.

Hill F. W. G. (1972) Malabsorption syndrome in the dog: a study of thirty-eight cases. *J. Small Anim. Pract.* **13**, 575.

Macartney L., Cornwell H. J. C., McCandlish I. A. P. and Thompson H. (1985) Isolation of a novel paramyxovirus from a dog with enteric disease. *Vet. Rec.* **117**, 205.

Quigley P. J. and Henry K. (1981) Eosinophilic enteritis in the dog: a case report with a brief review of the literature. *J. Comp. Path.* **91**, 387.

Simpson J. W. (1982) Bacterial overgrowth causing intestinal malabsorption in a dog. *Vet. Rec.* **110**, 335.

Weaver A. D. (1977) Canine intestinal intussusception *Vet. Rec.* **100**, 524.

Williams D. A. and Burrows C. F. (1981) Short bowel syndrome. *J. Small Anim. Pract.* **22**, 263.

Woods C. B., Pollock R. V. H. and Carmichael L. E. (1980) Canine parvoviral enteritis *J. Am. Anim. Hosp. Assoc.* **16**, 171.

Chapter 22

Disorders of the Large Intestine

1. Colitis/proctitis:
   a. Acute—aetiology similar to enteritis (Chapter 21):
      i. Bacterial infections—salmonellae, campylobacter?
      ii. Parasitic infections—*Trichuris vulpis*
                                protozoa (coccidia, giardia)
      iii. Foreign bodies (bones or needles).
   b. Chronic—aetiology uncertain:
      i. Idiopathic (ulcerative)—in many breeds
         —may become granulomatous? (serious—causes adhesions)
      ii. Histiocytic—in young Boxers (uncommon)
      iii. Eosinophilic—specific, or as in enteritis?
2. Neoplasia:
   a. Adenocarcinoma (malignant).
   b. Lymphosarcoma (malignant).
   c. Adenomatous polyp (benign).
   d. Leiomyoma (benign).
3. Stricture—unknown cause (may follow granulomatous colitis)
4. Constipation—usually secondary to:
   a. Prostatic disease (Chapter 30).
   b. Pelvic fracture.
   c. Spinal paralysis.
   d. Megacolon, colonic neoplasm, foreign body.
   e. Diet—low residue or bones.
   f. Pain (anal sacs, anal stricture, trauma).
   g. Laziness, debility, old age.
5. Megacolon—congenital or associated with:
   a. Perineal hernia
   b. Chronic infection.

6. 'Irritable colon syndrome' (psychological or stress?).
   —common in large dogs
   → intermittent and frequent defaecation.
7. Rectal prolapse.

Signs

    a. *Tenesmus* and frequency of defaecation.
    b. *Diarrhoea*—small quantities and frequently (except 4 and 5 *above*).
        Often with mucus and/or blood.

Findings

    a. Abdominal palpation occasionally reveals mass/pain/faecal concretions.
    b. Rectal examination frequently reveals the lesion (stricture, mega-colon, deviation, foreign body, neoplasm). Perineal hernia is also readily appreciated.

Investigations

    a. Faecal examination for parasites/bacteria/blood.
    b. Proctoscopy to identify lesion and for biopsy? (p. 141).
    c. Radiology (Chapter 35):
        i. Pneumocolography.
        ii. Barium meal or enema.

General therapy for diarrhoea (including diet)

See Chapter 23.

Specific therapy

    a. Colitis:
        i. Feed high-residue 'bulking' agents, e.g. bran.
        ii. Sulphasalazine (Salazopyrin; Pharmacia), 50 mg/kg/day reducing after 2 weeks to a *maximum* of 4 weeks
        iii. Antibiotics (tylosin) and corticosteroids (prednisolone)? *Only* for eosinophilic colitis or if no response to other therapy.

    b. Infections:
        i. Salmonellae—best *not* treated
            consider the public health risk.

    ii. Trichuris (*see* p. 129).
  c. Protozoa (*see* p. 129).
  d. Constipation and megacolon:
    i. 'Bulking' agents (bran).
    ii. Laxatives (Peridale; Dales or Visiblin; Parke Davis).
    iii. Manual relief.
    iv. Liquid paraffin?
  e. Other disorders—surgery may relieve:
    i. Neoplasms (can be resected or removed at proctoscopy?).
    ii. Strictures—or may be dilated manually.
    iii. Rectal prolapse.
  f. 'Irritable colon syndrome':
    i. High fibre diet (bran?)
    ii. Anticholinergics? (Atropine).
    iii. Opiates (loperamide; Imodium; diphenoxylate; Lomotil).

DIFFERENTIAL DIAGNOSIS OF ACUTE HAEMORRHAGIC DIARRHOEA

1. Haemorrhagic gastroenteritis (HGE).
2. Parvovirus infection.
3. Distemper infection.
4. Salmonella infection.
5. Coccidiosis.
6. Intussusception.
7. Colonic or rectal foreign body.
8. *Trichuris vulpis?*
9. Coagulopathies (Chapter 42).
10. Colitis.
11. Colonic or rectal neoplasm.
12. Other virus infections (including coronavirus)?

FURTHER READING

Ewing G. O. and Gomez J. A. (1973) Canine ulcerative colitis. *J. Am. Anim. Hosp. Assoc.* **9**, 395.

Lorenz M. D. (1983) Disorders of the large bowel. In: Ettinger S. J. (ed.), *Textbook of Veterinary Internal Medicine,* 2nd Ed. Philadelphia, Saunders.

Lorenz M. D. (1980) The management of colitis. In: Kirk R. W. (ed.), *Current Veterinary Therapy VII.* Philadelphia, Saunders.

Chapter 23

Differential Diagnosis and Management of Persistent Diarrhoea

Most cases of persistent or recurrent diarrhoea in dogs appear to be functional and they can often be resolved by symptomatic therapy.

Full investigation can be expensive.

The nature of faeces varies widely in normal dogs. Many large and giant breeds of dog rarely produce fully 'formed' faeces. Large dogs have a relatively small absorptive capacity compared with small dogs and some other species: they are often presented with persistent or recurrent diarrhoea.

Any disruption of small intestinal 'balance' may lead to diarrhoea:
1. Exosmosis (unabsorbed solute passes to the colon)
   (dietary overload/maldigestion/malabsorption)
   → increased liquids and fermentation in the colon.
   → inadequate water absorption in the colon.
2. Hypersecretion (exudation)
   (inflammation/enterotoxins/venous congestion)
   → increased volume to colon → inadequate water absorption.
3. Altered motility (increased, or loss of segmentation)
   (partial obstructions/malabsorption)
   → increased motility
   or stagnant bowel loop and bacterial overgrowth.

DIFFERENTIAL DIAGNOSIS

1. Incorrect or inappropriate diet
    a. Excesses, especially carbohydrates, fats.
    b. *Intolerance* (especially biscuits or meal).
    c. Scavenging—recurrent irritation.
    d. Allergies?

2. Maldigestion

- *a.* Pancreatic insufficiency (Chapter 27).
- *b.* Disaccharidase insufficiency (including lactase).
- *c.* Hepatic insufficiency or bile deficiency.
- *d.* Other brush border enzyme deficiencies?

3. Malabsorption

- *a.* Intestinal lymphosarcoma.
- *b.* Villous atrophy.
- *c.* Lymphangiectasia.
- *d.* Eosinophilic enteritis.
- *e.* Regional infiltrative enteritis
  (Lymphocytic, histiocytic, plasma cell or amyloid).
- *f.* Surgical resection.
- *g.* 'Carrier' failures.

4. Parasitic infection

- *a.* Nematodes (ascarids, Trichuris, Uncinaria).
- *b.* Protozoa (coccidia, Giardia).

5. Colonic irritation (*see* Chapter 22)

- *a.* Colitis.
- *b.* Foreign body.
- *c.* Adenocarcinoma.

6. Infection

- *a.* Salmonella, Campylobacter, Shigella?
- *b.* Distemper.
- *c.* Other viruses?
- *d.* Bacterial overgrowth within the gut.

7. Disorders of other systems

- *a.* Toxaemias (uraemia, hepatic failure, infections).
- *b.* Endocrine disturbances (diabetes mellitus, hypoadreno-corticalism, hyperthyroidism?, oestrus?).
- *c.* Congestive cardiac failure.

8. Psychological upsets

    a. Nervous dogs (e.g. German Shepherds).
    b. *Habit,* especially frequency—becomes behavioural?

9. Others

    a. Partially-obstructing, linear foreign body.
    b. Intussusception (partially-obstructing).
    c. Persistent use of antibiotic agents (especially neomycin).
       → bacterial overgrowth ± malabsorption.
    d. Stagnant bowel loop.

INVESTIGATION OF CHRONIC DIARRHOEA

1. History

    a. Feeding, diet, thirst.
    b. Duration, persistence, progression.
    c. Frequency of defaecation.
    d. Consistency of faeces.
    e. Colour of faeces.
    f. Presence of mucus or blood.
    g. Coprophagy (especially pancreatic insufficiency).
    h. Presence of other disease.
    i. General health.
N.B. If there is no weight loss and only variable diarrhoea, serious disease (e.g. malabsorption) is unlikely to be present.

2. Differentiation of region affected

    a. Small intestinal disorders:
       i. Occasional vomiting?
       ii. Weight loss.
       iii. Pale/fatty/watery/bulky faeces.
       iv. Flatulence or borborygmi.
       v. Diarrhoea a *few* times daily.
    b. Large intestinal disorders:
       i. Tenesmus and *frequency* (many times daily).
       ii. Small quantities of faeces passed.
       iii. Dark, jelly-like faeces, may be fresh blood and mucus.
       iv. (May be vomiting).

3. Findings

    a. Signs of other disorders:
       i. Endocrine? (Chapter 36).

    ii. Jaundice ? (Chapter 25).

    iii. Congestive cardiac failure?

  b. Mucous membranes—pallor?

    Lymph nodes—enlarged? (Lymphosarcoma?)

  c. Abdominal palpation:

    i. Foreign body, neoplasm?

    ii. Gas, bubblings in small intestines?

    iii. Pain?

  d. Rectal examination:

    i. Foreign body, neoplasm, lesions, ulceration?

    ii. Character of faeces?

MANAGEMENT OF CHRONIC DIARRHOEA

1. If signs suggest a disorder of the small intestine

a. Adjust the diet: initial action

    i. Starve for 24 hours of all food and milk.

    ii. Alter to bland food, e.g. lean mutton, tripe, chicken or cottage cheese with rice or potatoes.

    iii. Withdraw all milk, titbits and other foods (especially biscuits, fats, meal, liver, offal).

    iv. Keep from scavenging.

b. Check faecal sample for

    i. Parasites (or worm the dog with a broad-spectrum agent).

    ii. Undigested materials:

      Muscle fibres—if fed *raw* meat for 2 days.

      Starch granules—stain with Lugol's iodine.

      Fats—stain with Sudan IV.

        Globules: maldigestion?

        Unstained greasy material: malabsorption?

      Presence of these materials suggests malabsorption.

c. Collect fresh serial faecal samples for *trypsin digest test* (if signs suggest pancreatic insufficiency).

N.B. Interpret with care: if *serial samples* show consistently little activity, the cause *may* be pancreatic insufficiency *but* one or two low levels of faecal trypsin are of little significance.

d. Hospitalize if the problem persists and the cause is uncertain.

Many diarrhoeas (functional) will stop on admission.

If persistent diarrhoea:

i. Check:
   Consistency of faeces.
   Pattern of defaecation.
ii. Check haematology (anaemia, eosinophilia, leukaemia?).
iii. Check:
   Plasma urea (renal failure?).
   Liver enzymes (hepatic failure?).
   Cholesterol, calcium and proteins
   —may be low in maldigestion or malabsorption.
iv. Faecal culture (usually unhelpful).
v. Radiology and barium meal (Chapter 35) (not often helpful—may detect partially-obstructing foreign body, intussusception, neoplasia?).
vi. Serum folate and vitamin B_{12} levels may be altered (Batt and Morgan, 1982).
   Low B_{12} and *elevated* folate:
   (pancreatic insufficiency or bacterial overgrowth).
   Low B_{12} and folate (severe malabsorption).
   Low folates (proximal small intestinal malabsorption).
vii. *Fat assimilation test* (simple test):
   Starve the dog for 24 hours, pre-sample.
   Give 3 ml/kg body weight of corn oil.
   Re-sample at 2–4 hours for plasma turbidity and/or triglycerides.
   Raised in normal dogs (test one as a control?).
   No increase in maldigestion or malabsorption
   Can retest after mixing pancreatic extract with the cornoil—may help to identify pancreatic insufficiency.
viii. *Serum trypsin-like immunoreactivity* (Williams and Batt, 1983):
   Single blood sample, following overnight starvation.
   Possibly the most reliable test for pancreatic insufficiency.
ix. *Xylose absorption test* (Hill, Kidder and Frew, 1970):
   Starve the dog and pre-sample.
   Give 0·5 g/kg body weight of xylose (BDH) orally
   as 5 per cent solution (stomach tube).
   Take serial blood samples for xylose (½ hourly for 3 hours).
   Normal absorption gives $> 2·5$ mmol/l at 60–90 min (*Fig.* 8).
   Or *glucose absorption test* (less specific, but cheaper).
   Poor absorption indicates small intestinal disease (*Fig.* 9).

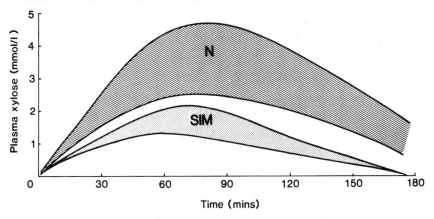

Fig. 8. Interpretation of the xylose absorption test (p. 138). Normal absorption usually produces a level >2·5 mmol/l at 60–90 min. N, range for normal dogs; SIM, small intestinal malabsorption.

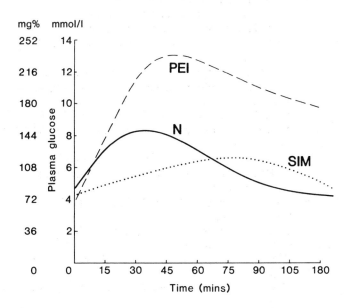

Fig. 9. Interpretation of the oral glucose absorption test. N, typical curve for normal dogs; PEI, typical curve in pancreatic exocrine insufficiency; SIM, typical curve in small intestinal malabsorption.

N.B. Tests affected by gastric emptying, renal excretion and bacterial overgrowth.

x. *Para-amino benzoic acid* (PABA) *test*
(Batt, Bush and Peters, 1979) (*Fig.* 10):
Starve dog for 24 hours, pre-sample.
Give 3·3 mmol/kg of PABA precursor (Fluorochem) as 0·33 mol/l solution in water at 10 ml/kg.
Sample for PABA at 30, 60, 90, 120, 240, 360 min.
See Fig. 10 for interpretation.
But may also be poor in slow gastric emptying or malabsorption.

xi. *Biopsy* following exploratory laparotomy or endoscopy (Johnson, 1980) may be the on way to *confirm* certain diagnoses (lymphosarcoma, villous atrophy, regional enteritis).
Duodenal juices may also be assessed for bacterial overgrowth, Giardia infection and enzyme assay.

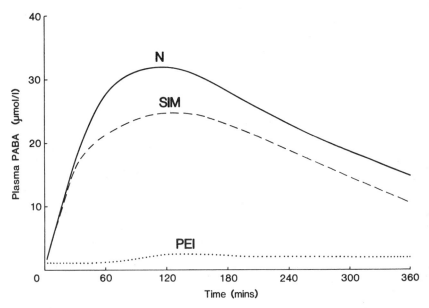

Fig. 10. Interpretation of the PABA test. N, typical curve for normal dogs; SIM, typical curve in small intestinal malabsorption; PEI typical curve in pancreatic exocrine insufficiency.

2. If signs suggest a disorder of the large intestine

  a. Re-check with a careful rectal examination.
  b. Radiology (Chapter 35):
    i. Plain film—foreign body neoplasia or partial obstruction?
    ii. Pneumocolography: inflate the colon via a tube with an inflatable cuff (relatively simple technique).
    iii. Following a barium enema.
    Following 24 hours' starvation and an enema, to empty the rectum.
  c. Proctoscopy.
    After 24 hours' starvation and an enema;
    a rigid or flexible fibreoptic endoscope may be used:
    i. To examine the mucosa (for ulceration, foreign body or neoplasia).
    ii. To take a biopsy of any lesion.

GENERAL MANAGEMENT FOR PERSISTENT DIARRHOEA

1. General

If the dog is well (with no weight loss, anaemia, or other signs suggesting malabsorption) and responds to hospitalization, suggesting an environmental or functional disturbance, but still has diarrhoea at home:

  a. Feed a bland diet (*see* p. 137).
  b. Add simple absorbants to food:
    i. Kaolin, bismuth, charcoal.
    ii. Peridale granules (Dales) or BCK granules (Loveridge).
  c. Try intestinal sedatives such as:
    i. Diphenoxylate (Lomotil; Searle) ($0.5–1.0$ mg/kg t.d.s.).
    ii. Loperamide (Immodium; Janssen) (1 or 2 daily to effect).
    iii. Chlorpromazine (if nervousness is a cause).
    iv. Aspirin (can reduce reaction to endotoxins).

2. Disorders of the small intestine (malabsorption)

  a. Diet: *see* p. 137.
    Additional readily-assimilated sources of energy include:
    i. Glucose.
    ii. Coconut oil (a medium-chain triglyceride).
  b. Oral corticosteroids (prednisolone 0.5 mg/kg/day, reducing): May be required for *proved* cases of regional enteritis or villous atrophy, may be aided by tylosin (40 mg/kg b.d.).

      c. Antibiotic therapy (e.g. oxytetracycline)—very few indications:
            i. Required for bacterial overgrowth or systemic infections.
           ii. Excessive use is very likely to alter flora, and *cause* problems.
      d. Vitamin supplementation
      Vitamin B and fat-soluble vitamins (e.g. Canovel; Beecham).

3. Pancreatic insufficiency—therapy is *expensive*

      a. i. Feed good quality protein (meat, e.g. tripe) and rice —little and often.
          ii. Feed no milk or conventional fats.
         iii. Feed glucose rather than starch.
      b. Add large quantities of pancreatic extract to food, before feeding (powdered preparation most effective e.g. Pancrex; Pabyrn).
      c. Give sodium bicarbonate or aluminium hydroxide or cimetidine (Tagamet; Smith Kline 10 mg/kg) ½ hour before feeding or with the food.
      d. Try feeding coconut oil as a separate meal.
      e. Vitamin supplementation (Canovel; Beecham) is advised.

REFERENCES AND FURTHER READING

Batt R. M. (1979) Technique for single and multiple peroral jejunal biopsy in the dog. *J. Small Anim. Pract.* **20**, 259.

Batt R. M. (1980) The molecular basis of malabsorption. *J. Small Anim. Pract.* **21**, 555.

Batt R. M. (1984) Chronic small intestinal disease in the dog. *J. Small Anim. Pract.* **25**, 707.

Batt R. M., Bush B. M. and Peters T. J. (1979) A new test for the diagnosis of exocrine pancreatic insufficiency in the dog. *J. Small Anim. Pract.* **20**, 185.

Batt R. M. and Mann L. C. (1981) The specificity of the BT-PABA Test for the diagnosis of exocrine pancreatic insufficiency in the dog. *Vet. Rec.* **108**, 303.

Batt R. M. and Morgan J. O. (1982) Role of serum folate and vitamin B_{12} concentrations in the differentiation of small intestinal abnormalities in the dog. *Res. Vet. Sci.* **32**, 17.

Burrows C. F., Merritt A. M. and Chiapella A. M. (1979) Determination of fecal fat and trypsin output in the evaluation of chronic canine diarrhoea. *J. Am. Vet. Med. Assoc.* **174**, 62.

Frankland A. L. (1969) An investigation of the trypsin digest test on apparently normal canine faeces. *J. Small Anim. Pract.* **10**, 531.

Hill F. W. G. (1972) Malabsorption syndrome in the dog: a study of thirty-eight cases. *J. Small Anim. Pract.* **13**, 575.

Hill F. W. G., Kidder D. E. and Frew J. (1970) A xylose absorption test for the dog. *Vet. Rec.* **87**, 250.

Johnson G. F. (1980) Duodenoscopy. In: Anderson N. V. (ed.), *Veterinary Gastroenterology*. Philadelphia, Lea & Febiger.

Pidgeon G. (1982) Effect of diet on exocrine pancreatic insufficiency in dogs. *J. Am. Vet. Med. Assoc.* **181**, 232.

Strombeck D. R. (1978) A new method for evaluation of chymotrypsin deficiency in dogs. *J. Am. Vet. Med. Assoc.* **173**, 1319.

van Kruiningen H. J. (1976) Clinical efficacy of tylosine in canine inflammatory bowel disease. *J. Am. Anim. Hosp. Assoc.* **12,** 498.

Willard M. D. (1985) Newer concepts in treatment of secretory diarrheas. *J. Am. Vet. Med. Assoc.* **186,** 86.

Williams D. A. and Batt R. M. (1983) Diagnosis of canine exocrine pancreatic insufficiency by the assay of serum trypsin-like immunoreactivity. *J. Small Anim. Pract.* **24,** 583.

Chapter 24

Hepatic Disorders

Signs of hepatic failure are often vague, and specific treatment is frequently impossible.

Problems associated with the ***diagnosis and management*** of hepatic disorders include:

1. The capacity of the liver for regeneration. In many instances, 80 per cent of hepatic tissue must lose function before the development of signs of failure. Degeneration and regeneration are often concurrent, causing variations in intensity of signs.
2. Clinical signs, apart from jaundice and ascites, are often vague. Even these signs require differentiation from other causes.
3. Liver enzymes do not accurately indicate the severity or type of hepatic disease. No single test specifies a lesion.
4. The liver is readily affected by other disease processes in the body, including cardiac failure, endocrine disorders and neoplasia, and it is readily damaged in the detoxification of poisons.

Hepatic functions include:

1. Synthesis of most plasma proteins (including albumin and the clotting factors).
2. Conversion of products of protein metabolism to urea.
3. Metabolism and storage of carbohydrates and fats.
4. Detoxification and excretion of poisons, drugs and hormones.
5. Production and excretion of bile.

The results of ***Chronic hepatic failure*** may therefore include:

1. Hypoproteinaemia ($\rightarrow$ ascites), coagulation disorders.
2. Hyperammonaemia and hepatic encephalopathy.
3. Weight loss, stunted growth, hyperlipidaemia, hypoglycaemia.

144

4. Toxaemia, excess aldosterone retention($\rightarrow$ ascites), abnormal drug metabolism.
5. Jaundice, maldigestion, pale faeces.
Additionally, there may be poor venous return to the heart
($\rightarrow$ ascites).

A. ACUTE HEPATIC DISORDERS (not common)

1. Infectious canine hepatitis:
   - *a.* Acute and severe $\rightarrow$ abdominal pain, shock (and sudden death).
   - *or* *b.* Mild $\rightarrow$ few hepatic signs
        (mild malaise, anorexia, digestive upset).
2. Leptospirosis.
3. Toxic hepatitis (probably uncommon)—agents include:
   - *a.* Poisons: glycol, carbon tetrachloride, tar, heavy metals, pesticides.
   - *b.* Drugs: primidone, phenytoin, phenothiazine derivatives, some steroids.
   - *c.* Endotoxins.
4. Hepatic trauma/rupture
   An occasional cause of haemorrhagic shock (Chapter 42).
5. Bile duct rupture causes *chronic* signs, especially jaundice and peritonitis.
6. (Other infections: salmonellosis, toxoplasmosis).
7. Acidophil cell hepatitis (Jarrett and O'Neil, 1985).

Signs

General signs are *non-specific:*
   - *a.* Anorexia, depression, lethargy.
   - *b.* Vomiting (not 4, 5), abdominal pain.

Findings (variable)

   - *a.* Pyrexia.
   - *b.* Jaundice (uncommon except with 2 or 5).
   - *c.* Petechial haemorrhages 1, 2.
   - *d.* Dark urine, pale faeces.
   - *e.* Occasionally: 'blue eye' on recovery, a few days later (1*b*).

Investigations (*see* Kelly, Lucke and Gaskell, 1982)

   - *a.* Liver enzymes:
      - i. GPT (ALT) is high (in 1, 2, 3, 7).
      - ii. Alkaline phosphatase may be elevated.

    b. Routine haematology:
       i. Haemolytic anaemia and leucocytosis (2).
       ii. Haemoconcentration and leucopenia (1*a*).
    c. Bilirubin—high levels may be found:
       i. Conjugated (5).
       ii. Unconjugated (2).
       iii. Mixed (1, 3).
    d. Serology (rising titres—1, 2).
    e. Liver biopsy may give a guide to diagnosis and prognosis (p. 151).

Treatment

See Acute Abdominal Disorders (Chapter 20).
    General Management for Hepatic Disorders (p.152).
Specifically: euthanasia for proven leptospirosis?
    (or administer high levels of penicillin and streptomycin).

Prognosis

Very guarded for most acute disorders, but if a dog survives the first few days, hepatic regeneration may permit full recovery.

B. CHRONIC HEPATIC DISORDERS

1. Primary neoplasia
    (haemangiosarcoma, hepatoma, bile duct tumours):
        Not as common as tumour metastases.
        May cause ascites (occasionally jaundice), bile duct obstruction.
2. Secondary neoplasia (haemangiosarcoma, lymphosarcoma, carcinomata, leukaemia, others)
3. Cirrhosis:
    a. Cause is usually unknown.
    b. Often accompanied by regeneration, but usually progressive.
    c. Ascites and/or jaundice are common.
4. Congenital lesions:
        Portosystemic anastomoses:
        may be primary or secondary to juvenile cirrhosis.
           Signs of hepatic failure at 6–9 months of age.
           Stunted growth and encephalopathy are common.
           Liver is usually small.
5. Chronic active hepatitis:
        Immune reaction to hepatitis virus or autoimmune disease.
        May result in cirrhosis.

6. Intrahepatic cholestasis:
   Other bile duct disorders (including cholelithiasis) are rare.
7. Amyloidosis (uncommon):
   Unknown aetiology—progressive.
   Other organs may be involved (kidneys, intestines).
8. Storage diseases/enzyme deficiencies (in young dogs)
   (including copper toxicosis in Bedlington terriers)

Signs

General signs are rather vague and *non-specific:*
   a. (Toxaemia):
      poor appetite, weight loss, depression, lethargy, variable vomiting.
   b. Sometimes: abdominal enlargement, polydipsia, pale faeces.
   c. Occasionally (variable signs): haemorrhages, diarrhoea, CNS disturbances, (encephalopathy): apathy, depression, aimless wandering, ataxia, seizures, stupidity, head pressing.

Findings

   a. Jaundice (especially with cirrhosis, cholestasis) ⎱ Variable.
   b. ?Ascites (especially with cirrhosis, neoplasia) ⎰
   c. Liver size:
      i. Enlarged with neoplasia.
      ii. Small with portosystemic shunts or cirrhosis.

Investigations

Laboratory tests:
   a. SGPT (ALT) is elevated in most disorders.
   b. Alkaline phosphatase is often markedly raised
      (up to 100 times normal).
   c. Any jaundice is hepatic or post-hepatic (bilirubin is elevated).
   d. Any ascitic fluid is a modified transudate (Chapter 34).
   e. Plasma proteins:
      albumin may be reduced; globulins may be elevated.
   f. Hypoglycaemia or hypercalcaemia is occasionally found.
   g. Clotting times may be prolonged.
   h. Serum cholesterol may be elevated.
   i. Biurate crystals may be present in urine ⎱ in hepatic
   j. Plasma ammonia is usually elevated   ⎰ encephalopathy.
   k. Plasma urea is usually depressed
   l. BSP retention is increased in most of these disorders.

Further investigations

    a. Radiography:
        i. Plain films.
    Unlikely to yield a specific diagnosis, but help to determine liver size and to identify neoplasia.
        ii. Contrast studies (Chapter 35):
    Splenic or mesenteric venous angiography is necessary to identify a portosystemic shunt.
    Cholecystography—for suspect biliary disorders.
    b. Exploratory laparotomy and/or biopsy.
        Objects:
        i. To confirm a diagnosis.
        ii. To aid prognosis and treatment.
        iii. To monitor progress.
    Repeat biopsies may be valuable to monitor progress.
    c. Biopsy can be obtained without general anaesthesia (p. 151).

Specific treatment

    a. Potentially possible partially to occlude portocaval shunts with materials that bind slowly. (Breznock *et al,* 1983).
    b. Chronic active hepatitis may respond to corticosteroid therapy.
    Most other lesions are potentially fatal—euthanasia is advised.

General management *see* p. 152

Prognosis

Guarded or hopeless for most of these disorders.
It may be indicated by changes in biochemical test results.

C. OTHER DISORDERS AFFECTING THE LIVER

Occur commonly, particularly causing *hepatic enlargement.*
1. Chronic venous congestion due to:
    a. Right-sided or congestive cardiac failure.
    b. Neoplastic obstruction of great veins.
    Liver enzymes are usually slightly raised (to five times normal).
    BSP retention is increased.
2. Fatty degeneration/infiltration.
    Usually due to metabolic or endocrine disorders:
    a. Diabetes mellitus.
    b. Hyperadrenocorticalism.

   c. Hypothyroidism.
   d. Hyperlipidosis.
Liver enzymes markedly are raised, especially alkaline phosphatase.
These disorders may be reversible, but may progress to cirrhosis.
3. Extrahepatic biliary obstruction:
   a. Pancreatic adenocarcinoma or pancreatitis.
   b. Intestinal neoplasia or obstruction.
   c. (Gallstones) *rare.*
   d. Bile duct neoplasia.
High levels of conjugated bilirubin and alkaline phosphatase.
(An indication for exploratory laparotomy.)

DIAGNOSIS OF HEPATIC DISORDERS
(*see* Kelly, Lucke and Gaskell, 1982)

1. Liver enzymes

Problems
   i. *Not* specific for a particular type of disease.
   ii. Dozens are used in man, indicating lack of specificity.
   iii. Often raised in other generalized diseases.
   iv. Levels vary considerably from day to day.
  a. *Serum glutamic pyruvic transamonase* (SGPT)
   (alanine aminotransferase: ALT) (Normal level:
   10–20 i.u./l):
     i. Fairly specific for hepatocellular damage (necrosis or
      inflammation).
     ii. Very readily released even by insignificant disease,
      elevated in many acute hepatic disorders and with excess
      glucocorticoids.
     iii. Very high in hepatitis ($10 \times$ normal).
     iv. Levels are not as high in most chronic disorders.
  b. *Serum glutamic oxaloacetic transaminase* (SGOT)
   (aspartate aminotransferase:AST):
   Also released in hepatocellular damage, but it is present in
   significant quantitites in other body tissues in small animals.
  c. *Serum alkaline phosphatase* (SAP) (Normal level: 3–15 K.A.
   units):
     i. Enzyme found in a number of tissues (e.g. bone and
      kidney).
     ii. Normally excreted in bile.
     iii. Released in large quantities when bile ducts are
      obstructed.
     iv. Raised by many hepatic or post-hepatic disorders (in
      cholestasis).

      v. Levels are especially high (10 × to 100 × normal) with hepatic cirrhosis, fatty degeneration, neoplasia, cholestasis and post-hepatic obstruction.

     vi. Consistently high levels are a reliable indication for exploratory laparotomy and/or biopsy.

  d. Others:

     i. Sorbitol dehydrogenase (SDH).

    ii. Lactic dehydrogenase (LDH).

   iii. Gamma glutamyl transferase (γGT).

  Can also be employed in dogs, but of little additional value.

2. Liver function

  a. Bilirubin may be elevated by:

     i. Excess haemolysis

       → unconjugated (indirect-reacting Van den Bergh)

    ii. Failure of hepatic conjugation

      (e.g. neoplasia, cirrhosis, hepatitis)→ mixed reaction.

   iii. Impaired excretion of bilirubin

      → conjugated (direct-reacting Van den Bergh)

      (e.g. bile duct obstruction or rupture).

Total serum bilrubin is composed of conjugated bilirubin, direct-reacting to Van den Bergh's Test and unconjugated bilirubin (indirect-reacting). The proportions indicated the source (p. 155). Quite useful in monitoring the course and progress of disease.

  b. Bromsulphthalein (BSP) excretion/retention:

    5 mg/kg b.w. of this dye are injected intravenously. A blood sample 30 minutes later should reveal only 5 per cent retention.

    The test is influenced by circulatory function, but excessive retention of BSP is fairly reliable evidence of serious hepatic dysfunction.

3. Other tests

  a. Plasma proteins

     i. Plasma albumin levels become depressed in chronic hepatic disorders although not as markedly as in some other species.

    ii. Gamma globulin levels are often elevated, so that total protein levels may remain normal.

   iii. Plasma clotting factors may be depressed, with prolonged prothrombin and clotting times, especially in chronic disorders.

b. Plasma cholesterol
Levels may rise, especially in obstructive disorders in glucocorticoid excess and in hypoalbuminaemia.

c. Other findings Many other tests can be applied.

Plasma ammonia may be high ⎫ in hepatic encephalopathy
Plasma urea may be depressed ⎰ (e.g. portosystemic shunts)

An *ammonia tolerance test* may be employed (Meyer *et al,* 1978).
Plasma glucose levels may be slightly raised or depressed.

Urinalysis:
- i.   Bilirubinuria may occur especially in obstructive jaundice, but it is present in many *normal* dogs.
- ii. Bile pigments (urobilin) may be present in prehepatic jaundice.
- iii. Bile salts may be present in biliary obstruction.
- iv. Biurate crystals may be found with hyperammonaemia.

4. Other investigations

a. Radiography
This is an important aid to the diagnosis of hepatic size and the presence of any masses, but is unlikely to yield a specific diagnosis. The position of the stomach gas shadow is a good indicator of the size of the liver. Cholecystography has been successfully employed in small animals but there are few indications for this technique (Chapter 35).
Care is essential with any anaesthesia:
- i. Minimize quantities.
- ii. Avoid phenothiazines and halothane.

b. Exploratory laparotomy and/or biopsy
These are the only means of confirming a diagnosis and giving indications for treatment and prognosis in many cases.
Biopsy technique (Chapman, 1965):
- i.   Local anaesthesia and aseptic precautions.
- ii. Small skin incision between xiphoid and last rib.
- iii. Another incision for finger of a gloved hand to stabilize the *left* liver lobe and to avoid the gallbladder.
- iv. Insert a Tru-cut needle (Travenol), biopsy and withdraw (Angle the needle 20° leftwards, 20° forwards and dorsally).

GENERAL MANAGEMENT OF HEPATIC DISEASE AND FAILURE

Removal of the causal agent is not often possible.

Little specific therapy is available—much is supportive and symptomatic.
Optimum facilities for hepatic regeneration should be provided.

1. Therapeutic measures

    a. Cage rest—to minimize discomfort and demands on the liver
    b. Dietary management:
       Oral feeding is often poorly tolerated in acute failure
       —intravenous therapy may be needed.
       i. Calorie intake should be kept as high as possible
          —in the form of carbohydrates (rice, sugar, starch).
       ii. Fat intake should be minimized.
       iii. Protein intake (of good quality) should be maintained
          (e.g. canned rice, eggs, cottage cheese and meat).
          (*Unless* signs of CNS dysfunction are seen— see *3d* below.)
       iv. Generally—low residue and low salt are also required.
    c. Supportive treatment:
       i. Use anabolic steroids to discourage catabolism.
       ii. Supplement vitamins B, C, K and zinc.
       iii. The addition of choline and methionine (lipotrophics) is of doubtful value in fatty liver.
       iv. Pancreatic extract and bile salts (Panteric; Parke Davis) may help if there is any evidence of maldigestion.
       v. If hepatic encephalopathy occurs:
       Protein intake should be minimized (and of high quality).
       Oral administration of neomycin (20 mg/kg t.i.d.) and of lactulose (Duphalac; Duphar) (5–30 ml t.i.d.) may help to minimize the absorption of toxic agents from the gut.
    d. Other drugs:
       i. Tetracyclines are metabolized and excreted by the liver, and are therefore valuable for hepatic disorders, but levels may build up excessively in hepatic failure. Ampicillin and erythromycin are also excreted by the liver.
       ii. Phenothiazine derivatives such as acetylpromazine should be avoided, also benzodiazepines (e.g. diazepam).
       iii. Anticonvulsants (phenytoin, primidone) are metabolized by the liver. Normal therapeutic levels may cause toxicity in hepatic failure.
       iv. Potentially hepatotoxic agents such as halothane should not be employed.
       v. Corticosteroids may have beneficial effects in some cases of hepatic failure (e.g. chronic active hepatitis). They are otherwise undesirable.

    e. Diuresis may be required for the treatment of ascites. It is certainly preferable to repeated paracentesis.

DIFFERENTIAL DIAGNOSIS OF HEPATOMEGALY

1. Raised venous pressure, congestion:
    a. Congestive or right-sided cardiac failure.
    b. Neoplastic obstruction of venous return to the heart.
2. Fatty infiltration:
    a. Obesity.
    b. Diabetes mellitus.
    c. Hyperadrenocorticalism.
    d. Hypothyroidism.
    e. Toxic hepatitis.
    f. Hyperlipidosis.
3. Neoplasia:
    a. Primary hepatoma.
    b. Generalized lymphosarcoma.
    c. Haemangiosarcoma.
    d. Metastases (carcinomata).
    e. Leukaemias.
4. Other disorders:
    a. Hepatitis.
    b. Amyloidosis.
    c. Biliary obstruction?
    d. Autoimmune haemolytic anaemia.

REFERENCES AND FURTHER READING

Breznock E. M. (1979) Surgical manipulation of portosystemic shunts in dogs. *J. Am. Vet. Med. Assoc.* **174,** 819.

Breznock E. M., Berger B., Pendray D., Wagner S., Manley P., Whiting P., Hornof W. and West D. (1983) Surgical manipulation of intrahepatic portocaval shunts in dogs. *J. Am. Vet. Med. Assoc.* **182,** 798.

Bunch S. E., Castleman W. L., Hornbuckle W. E. and Tennant B. C. (1982) Hepatic cirrhosis associated with long-term anticonvulsant drug therapy in dogs. *J. Am. Vet. Med. Assoc.* **181,** 357.

Bush B. M. (1980) The laboratory evaluation of canine hepatic disease. In: Grunsell C. S. G. and Hill F. W. G. (ed.), *Veterinary Annual.* Bristol, Wright Scientechnica.

Chapman W. L. (1965) Liver biopsy in the dog. *J. Am. Vet. Med. Assoc.* **146,** 126.

Cornelius C. E. (1979) Biochemical evaluation of hepatic function in dogs. *J. Am. Anim. Hosp. Assoc.* **15,** 259.

Doige D. E. and Lester S. (1981) Chronic active hepatitis in dogs. A review of fourteen cases. *J. Am. Anim. Hosp. Assoc.* **17,** 725.

Feldman E. C. and Ettinger S. J. (1979) Percutaneous transthoracic liver biopsy in the dog. *J. Am. Vet. Med. Assoc.* **169,** 805.

Jarrett W. F. H. and O'Neil B. W. (1985) A new transmissable agent causing acute hepatitis, chronic hepatitis and cirrhosis in dogs. *Vet. Rec.* **116,** 629.

Kelly D. F., Lucke V. M. and Gaskell C. J. (1982) *Notes on Pathology for Small Animal Clinicians.* Bristol, Wright PSG.

Maddison J. E. (1981) Portosystemic encephalopathy in two young dogs: some additional diagnostic and therapeutic considerations. *J. Small Anim. Pract.* **22**, 731.

McConnell M. F. and Lumsden J. H. (1983) Evaluation of metastatic liver disease in the dog. *J. Am. Anim. Hosp.* **19**, 173.

Meyer D. J., Stombeck D. R., Stone E. A., Zenoble R. D. and Buss D. D. (1978) Ammonia tolerance test in clinically normal dogs and in dogs with portosystemic shunts. *J. Am. Vet. Med. Assoc.* **173**, 377.

Milne E. M. (1985) The diagnostic value of alkaline phosphatase in canine medicine: a review. *J. Small Anim. Pract.* **26**, 267.

Mullowney P. C. and Tennant B. C. (1982) Choledocolithiasis in the dog; a review and a report of a case with rupture of the common bile duct. *J. Small Anim. Pract.* **23**, 631.

Murdoch D. B. (1978) Treatment of hepatic disease in small animals. In: Grunsell C. S. G. and Hill F. W. G. (ed.) *Veterinary Annual.* Bristol, Wright Scientechnica.

Murdoch D. B. (1980) Clinical features of liver disease in the dog. In: Grunsell C. S. G. and Hill F. W. G. (ed.), *Veterinary Annual.* Bristol, Wright Scientechnica.

Osborne C. A., Stevens J. B. and Perman V. (1969) Needle biopsy of the liver. *J. Am. Vet. Med. Assoc.* **155**, 1605.

Rothuizen J., van den Ingh Th. S. G. A. M., Voorhout G. et al. (1982) Congenital portosystemic shunts in sixteen dogs and three cats. *J. Small Anim. Pract.* **23**, 67.

Strombeck D. R. (1978) Clinicopathologic features of primary and metastatic neoplasia of the liver in dogs. *J. Am. Vet. Med. Assoc.* **173**, 267.

Strombeck D. R. and Gribble D. (1978) Chronic active hepatitis in the dog. *J. Am. Vet. Med. Assoc.* **173**, 380.

Strombeck D. R., Weiser M. G. and Kaneko J. J. (1975) Hyperammonemia and hepatic encephalopathy in the dog. *J. Am. Vet. Med. Assoc.* **166**, 1105.

Twedt D. C. (1981) Jaundice, hepatic trauma and hepatic encephalopathy. *Vet. Clin. N. Am.* **11**, 121.

Twedt D. C., Sternlieb I. and Gilbertson S. R. (1979) Clinical, morphologic and chemical studies on copper toxicosis of Bedlington terriers. *J. Am. Vet. Med. Assoc.* **175**, 269.

Watkins P. E., Pearson H. and Denny H. R. (1983) Traumatic rupture of the bile duct in the dog: a report of seven cases. *J. Small Anim. Pract.* **24**, 731.

Chapter 25

Differential Diagnosis and Investigation of Jaundice

Staining of tissues with bilirubin—not always related to plasma levels. Jaundice does *not* always indicate hepatic disease.

Bilirubin (normal level<$6\cdot8\mu$mol/l;<2 mg per cent) is:

a. A product of breakdown of haemoglobin (spleen, RE system).
b. Circulated → liver (alcohol-soluble bilirubin).
c. Converted (conjugated) → water-soluble (by the liver).
d. Excreted → bile duct → intestine.
e. Converted in intestines → stercobilin → brown faeces.

1. Prehepatic jaundice (unconjugated, indirectly-reacting bilirubin)
Due to *haemolysis* (jaundice occurs when the liver is overloaded.

a. *Autoimmune haemolytic anaemia* (Chapter 40):
(Not commonly causing jaundice or haemoglobinuria in dogs.)
→ Severe and highly regenerative anaemia (Chapter 42).
b. *Incompatible blood transfusions* (Chapter 42):
  i. Sixty per cent of dogs are A +ve (universal recipients).
  ii. Transfusion reaction is not as powerful as in man.
  iii. Only subsequent incompatible transfusions cause haemolysis.
c. *Other:*
  i. Congenital haemolysis, e.g. Basenjis.
  ii. Acceleration of the natural process of haemolysis at the end of red cell life span can occur in many disorders, e.g. renal failure, sepsis.

    iii. Leptospirosis.
    iv. Leishmaniasis, haemobartonellosis, babesiasis (imported dogs).
N.B. Bilirubin becomes conjugated after a few days.

2. 'Hepatic' jaundice (mixed conjugated and unconjugated)
(Liver enzymes also generally high.)
    a. (Viral hepatitis), leptospirosis.
    b. Cirrhosis, neoplasia, amyloidosis.
    c. Toxic hepatitis.
    d. Chronic active hepatitis.
    e. Intrahepatic cholestasis.
    f. (Salmonellosis, toxoplasmosis).

3. 'Post-hepatic' jaundice (mainly conjugated, directly-reacting bilirubin)
    i. Alkaline phosphatase may also be very high.
    ii. Excess urinary excretion of bilirubin—pale faeces.
    iii. Usually indicates *biliary obstruction*.
    a. Neoplasia of:
        i. Pancreas (region of bile duct).
        ii. Bile duct.
        iii. Duodenal opening.
    b. Ruptured bile duct.
    c. Pancreatitis.
    d. Gallstones or other bile duct obstruction, cholangitis.
    e. Duodenal obstruction.

Investigations

    a. Test the plasma for bilirubin (and Van den Bergh test)—conjugated or unconjugated bilirubin?
    b. Check the urine for urobilin (high in haemolysis).
    Check for pale faeces and high fat content
    (indicate obstructive jaundice).
    c. Check routine haematology—haemolysis and regeneration? (Chapter 42).
    d. Check liver enzymes—hepatic or other disease?
    e. Consider cholecystography in post-hepatic jaundice (Chapter 35).
    f. Exploratory laparotomy is strongly indicated in most cases of post-hepatic jaundice. Biopsy may be necessary.

FURTHER READING

Murdoch D. B. (1976) Jaundice in the dog. *J. Small Anim. Pract.* **17**, 119.

Chapter 26

Splenic Disorders

N.B. Gross day-to-day variations in size occur, e.g.:
1. Enlargement with barbiturate anaesthesia.
2. Contraction with exercise or haemorrhage.

Disorders

　　a. Neoplasia:
　　　　i. Lymphosarcoma—diffuse enlargement.
　　　　ii. Haemangioma or haemangiosarcoma.
　　　　May rupture to cause repeated abdominal haemorrhage.
　　　　Especially common in German Shepherd dogs.
　　　　iii. Carcinomata, sarcomata occasionally metastasize.
　　　　iv. Leukaemias.
　　b. Hyperplasia:
　　　　Benign nodular hyperplasia is common and easily confused
　　　　with neoplasia. Hyperplasia also occurs in haemolysis.
　　c. Splenomegaly may indicate other disease, e.g.:
　　　　i. Venous congestion (congestive or right-sided cardiac
　　　　　failure).
　　　　ii. Autoimmune disorders (Chapter 40)
　　　　　—haemolytic anaemia; thrombocytopenia.
　　　　iii. Other anaemias (Chapter 42).
　　　　iv. Infections (viral/bacterial).
　　　　v. Leukaemias.
　　　　vi. Idiopathic enlargement also occurs.
　　d. Torsion (causes acute abdominal pain, vomiting,
　　　depression).

    e. Amyloidosis.
    f. Haematoma.
Few *specific* signs of splenic disease are usually to be found.

Findings

    a. Palpable when enlarged.
    b. Usually obvious on radiographs enlarged in torsion.
    c. Exploratory laparotomy and histopathology *might* be indicated
       in case of doubt about diagnosis.

Treatment

Splenectomy:
    a. Is indicated in torsion.
    b. May be indicated in recurrent or persistent enlargement (*c*ii
       above) for torsion or for neoplasia.

FURTHER READING

Brown N. O., Patnaik A. K. and MacEwen E. G. (1985) Canine hemangiosarcoma: retrospective analysis of 104 cases *J. Am. Vet. Med. Assoc.* **186,** 56.
Feldman B. F. and Zinkl J. G. (1983) Diseases of the lymph nodes and spleen. In: Ettinger S. J. (ed.), *Textbook of Veterinary Internal Medicine,* 2nd Ed. Philadelphia, Saunders.
Frey A. J. and Betts C. W. (1977) A retrospective study of splenectomy in the dog. *J. Am. Anim. Hosp. Assoc.* **13,** 730.
Ishmael J. McC. and Howel J. (1968) Neoplasia of the spleen of the dog with a note on nodular hyperplasia. *J. Comp. Path.* **78,** 59.
Stead A. C., Frankland A. L. and Borthwick R. (1983) Splenic torsion in dogs. *J. Small Anim. Pract.* **24,** 549.
Stevenson S., Chew D. J. and Kociba G. J. (1981) Torsion of the splenic pedicle in the dog: a review. *J. Am. Anim. Hosp. Assoc.* **17,** 239.

Chapter 27

Pancreatic Disorders

A. PANCREATIC EXOCRINE INSUFFICIENCY

Aetiology

    a. Pancreatic degenerative atrophy:
        Usually occurs in young dogs (1–2 years old)
        especially German Shepherds and Collies.
    b. Fibrosis (following necrosis or recurrent pancreatitis?).
    c. Neoplasia or obstruction to the bile duct.
    d. Inactivation of pancreatic enzymes?
    e. Pancreatic hypoplasia?

Signs

    a. Dogs develop well, then lose weight, despite insatiable
        appetite.
    b. Pale voluminous rancid faeces or yellow diarrhoea.
    c. Coprophagy is common.

Diagnosis and treatment *See* Chronic Diarrhoea (Chapter 23).

B. PANCREATIC NECROSIS (PANCREATITIS)

Usually occurs in overweight middle-aged dogs, especially following a fatty meal. Pancreatic duct obstruction or reflux?
Necrosis and autolysis of pancreatic tissue cause haemorrhage, inflammation, oedema in connective tissues and fat necrosis → peritonitis, severe abdominal pain and *shock* with electrolyte loss and ileus.

159

May cause disseminated intravascular coagulation (DIC—*see* Chapter 42).

Signs

Acute depression, collapse and abdominal pain (praying stance?), anorexia, vomiting (mucus/bile). Sometimes dyspnoea.

Findings

    a. Pale mucous membranes, dehydration.
    b. May be haemorrhages
    c. Pyrexia.
    d. Pulse is rapid and weak and often irregular.
    e. Anterior abdominal pain.

Investigations

    a. Very high plasma amylase and lipase for up to 5 days (10 × normal).
    b. Leucocytosis, prerenal uraemia, hyperglycaemia, hypocalcaemia haemoconcentration, raised liver enzyme levels, electrolyte imbalance, DIC and hyperlipidaemia may all be found.
    c. Barium contrast radiography: static duodenal loop?
    d. Abdominal paracentesis → serosanguineous fluid.

Differential diagnosis and management

For details *see* Chapter 20.

Specific treatment

    a. *Starvation* for 2–4 days.
    b. *Drugs:*
        i. Intravenous fluids: plasma substitute (Haemaccel; Hoechst) then Ringer's lactate and bicarbonate and warmth.
        ii. Pethidine (4 mg/kg body weight i.m.).
        iii. Atropine (0·3–1·0 mg s.c.).
        iv. Corticosteroids and antibiotics.
        v. Glucagon (Lilly) (0·5–1·0 mg i.v. t.d.s.).
    c. Laparotomy and resection, following fluid therapy? (Denny and Lucke, 1972).
    d. Keep off fatty foods and reduce body weight if obese?

Consequences

- *a.* May result in fibrosis and exocrine and/or endocrine insufficiency.
- *b.* Not much evidence of recurrent pancreatitis in dogs.

C. NEOPLASIA (adenocarcinoma: in old dogs)

Signs

- *a.* General debilitating signs of neoplasia:
  weight loss, poor appetite, over weeks or months.
- *b.* Post-hepatic jaundice, due to bile duct obstruction (Chapter 25).
- c. Pancreatic exocrine insufficiency.
- *d.* Diabetes mellitus (uncommon).

Findings

- *a.* Occasionally palpable as an anterior abdominal mass.
- *b.* Radiography (with barium contrast or cholecystography) may reveal an anterior abdominal mass (Chapter 35).
- *c.* Plasma amylase and lipase are usually normal, but levels of alkaline phosphatase and conjugated bilirubin may be raised.
- *d.* Specific diagnosis is usually only possible by laparotomy and biopsy.

Treatment

Usually not possible—malignant.

D. DIABETES MELLITUS

See Chapter 36.

E. ISLET CELL TUMOUR

See Chapter 36.

REFERENCES AND FURTHER READING

Denny H. R. and Lucke J. N. (1972) A case of acute pancreatic necrosis in the dog. *J. Small Anim. Pract.* **13**, 545.

Hill F. W. G. (1978) Pancreatic disorders of dogs. In: Grunsell C. S. G. and Hill F. W. G. (ed.), *Veterinary Annual*. Bristol, Wright Scientechnica.

Hill F. W. G., Osborne A. D. and Kidder D. E. (1971) Pancreatic degenerative atrophy in dogs. *J. Comp. Path.* **81**, 321.

Schaer M. (1979) A clinicopathologic survey of acute pancreatitis in 30 dogs and 5 cats *J. Am. Anim. Hosp. Assoc.* **15**, 681.

Chapter 28

Renal Disorders

Signs of *disease* are usually noticed only when renal *failure* develops, following the loss of function of more than two-thirds of nephrons.

Clinically recognizable syndromes include:
1. Acute renal failure.
2. Chronic renal failure.
3. Nephrotic syndrome.

There may be a suspicion of the presence of other *disease* in the absence of renal *failure,* e.g.:
1. Neoplasia (palpable or seen on radiographs)—*rare.*
2. Pyelonephritis (pyuria, haematuria, pyrexia).
3. Renal calculi (radiographic finding)—uncommon.
4. Hydronephrosis (urinary obstruction—radiographic finding).
5. Trauma.

A. ACUTE RENAL FAILURE

Aetiology
> *a.* Tubular failure—may be due to:
>> i. Severe dehydration, circulatory failure, hypovolaemia.
>> ii. Poisoning—aminoglycosides, sulphonamides, ethylene glycol, paraquat, heavy metals.
>> iii. Vascular obstruction, ischaemia, hypercalcaemia.
> *b.* Acute interstitial nephritis (including leptospirosis).

    c. Glomerular failure:
        i. May be due to immune reaction to infection.
        ii. Autoimmune disease.
        iii. Toxaemic damage (especially pyometra or sepsis).
    d. Urinary tract obstruction (trauma, calculi, tumour).
    e. Urinary retention in the bladder.
    f. Trauma
    g. Acute diffuse pyelonephritis.
    h. Decompensating chronic renal disease.

Signs

Those of an acute abdominal crisis:
    a. Depression, anorexia, vomiting, abdominal pain.
    b. Initial oliguria (may → polyuria later).

Findings

Congested mucous membranes, dehydration, pain over kidneys?
Variable pyrexia, or hypothermia, tachycardia.

Laboratory findings

    a. Plasma urea rises fast (urea>40 mg per cent; >8 mmol/l).
    b. Plasma potassium rises.
    c. Urine:
        i. S.g. may be high initially, then may fall.
        ii. Many casts may be present.
        iii. Blood and protein may be present.
    d. Renal biopsy may give a guide to:
        i. Prognosis—some disorders may be *reversible*.
        ii. Definitive diagnosis.

Treatment

Acute renal failure is a potentially reversible disorder.
    a. Consider the cause—is specific therapy indicated?
    b. Restore the circulating volume and counteract dehydration
       (normal saline i.v.).
    c. Attempt to 're-open' kidneys with osmotic diuresis
       (20–50 ml/kg body weight of 10–20 per cent glucose i.v.).
    d. Consider peritoneal dialysis while awaiting re-function
       (Jackson, 1964).

    e. Supportive therapy: warmth, antiemetics, B vitamins, antibiotics?

    f. Monitor plasma urea and urine output
      —improvement may indicate a more favourable prognosis.

Fluid therapy should be withheld if no urine is produced, but acute renal failure may be reversible if fluid therapy is effective.

B. CHRONIC RENAL FAILURE (fibrotic 'end-stage' kidneys)

Aetiology

    a. Congenital dysplasias (esp. cocker spaniel, wheaten terrier).
    b. Chronic interstitial nephritis (leptospirosis? adenovirus?).
    c. Glomerulonephritis (especially fibrinous).
    d. Neoplasia.
    e. Pyelonephritis (generalized).
    f. Amyloidosis (progressive).
    g. Hydronephrosis.

Effects

    a. Inability to concentrate urine → loss of fluids → *polydipsia*.
    b. Catabolism of body tissues and toxaemia → *weight loss*.
    c. Retention of waste products (e.g. urea, creatinine, guanidine, phenols, uric acid, phosphates and potassium) → *toxaemia*.
    d. Increased RBC fragility, toxaemic marrow depression, alimentary haemorrhage and lack of erythropoietin → *anaemia*.
    e. Hyperparathyroidism → bone resorption (*rubber jaw*).

Signs (very variable)

    a. Compensated: remaining nephrons may increase fluid output → insidious polydipsia, polyuria.
    b. Decompensating uraemia (toxaemia):
      remaining nephrons can no longer clear wastes → polydipsia, polyuria, weight loss, anorexia, vomiting, depression, halitosis.

Findings (very variable)

    a. Ulcerated mucous membranes, anaemia, dehydration.
    b. Osteodystrophia fibrosa ('rubber jaw').
    c. Hard pulse.
    d. Shrunken and knobbly kidneys.
    e. Finally, convulsions, muscle twitch and coma may be seen.

Laboratory findings

   a. Blood:
- i. Anaemia (non-regenerative) lymphopenia are common.
- ii. Urea rises from normal (>40 mg per cent; >8 mmol/l).
- iii. Creatinine, inorganic phosphate levels rise.
- iv. Potassium rises and calcium falls *late* in disease.

   b. Urine:
- i. S.g. is low—usually at fixation point ($1\cdot008$–$1\cdot015$).
- ii. Urea level<20 g/l.
- iii. *Inability* to concentrate urine (Chapter 38).
- iv. Protein level is usually fairly *low.*
- v. Casts are variably found. Glycosuria occurs occasionally.
- vi. Urine: plasma urea ratio $<20:1$.

   c. Various clearance tests are available (sodium sulfanilate, inulin creatinine).

   d. Biopsy is the only means of confirming irreversibility.

Treatment

Treatment must be aimed towards avoidance of decompensation. The prognosis is ultimately grave, but signs may be relieved for a while. Client information and education is important.

   a. General aims:
- i. Replace loss of body fluids and electrolytes.
- ii. Encourage excretion of waste products.
- iii. Discourage formation of waste products.

   b. Water must be freely available at all times (if retained). Fluid losses in dehydration must be replaced (normal saline intravenously).

   c. *Rest* is important, and stress should be avoided.

   d. Food:
- i. Proteins:
  Reduce to a minimum but of high quality. Eggs and meat rather than offal or vegetable. 2 g/kg body weight daily *maximum* is advised.
- ii. Carbohydrates and fats should be plentiful. Rice and pasta are preferable to cereals, meal and biscuits.
- iii. Suggestions—feed little and often:
  Eggs, cottage cheese, meat and cooked rice, pasta.
  Tinned rice pudding and sugar.
  Tinned nephritis diet.
  Flavourings, e.g. Marmite.
  For energy: corn oil, butter, glucose, sugar.

   e. Aluminium hydroxide (Mucaine; Wyeth) may be administered
      orally: (reduces vomiting and absorption of phosphates)
         Cimetidine (Tagamet; Smith, Kline) may help in gastric
      ulceration
   f. Anabolic steroids should be used regularly:
       i. Reduce catabolism of tissues and R.B.C. fragility.
      ii. Encourage appetite and haemopoiesis.
   g. Replace sodium loss, encourage thirst and minimize acidosis.
      Sodium bicarbonate 30 mg/kg/day in divided doses.
   h. Supportive therapy as for acute renal failure (Chapter 28).
      Be very careful with drugs—may accumulate.

C. NEPHROTIC SYNDROME

An oedematous disorder due to gross protein loss through the
glomeruli.

Causes

   a. Immunologically-mediated damage to glomerular basement
      membrane (infections or autoimmune disorders).
   b. Amyloidosis.
Glomerular damage may be a common day-to-day occurrence, often
with no clinical significance unless the kidneys are severely affected.

Signs

   a. Subcutaneous oedema, ascites (± dyspnoea).
   b. Some weight loss, exercise intolerance.
   c. The dog may be quite bright and active, unless uraemic.
   d. May or may not be uraemic—if so, then signs are those of
      decompensated chronic renal failure.

Findings

   a. Generalized subcutaneous oedema.
   b. Pleural effusion, ascites.

Investigations

   a. Plasma protein levels below 50 g/l (albumin <20 g/l).
   b. Elevated plasma cholesterol is usual.
   c. Proteinuria very heavy (>10 g/l).
   d. Urine casts may be present.

e. Effusions are true transudates, with little protein content (Chapter 7).

f. Plasma urea, phosphates may rise
g. Urine concentration may fall. } if uraemia develops.

h. Biopsy is required for prognosis and definitive diagnosis.

Treatment

In the absence of uraemia, some of the treatment is at variance with that required for chronic renal failure:

a. *High* protein, salt-*free* diet is required (but monitor blood urea).

b. B vitamins and anabolic steroids should be administered, as in chronic renal failure.

c. Diuresis is indicated to reduce oedema and effusions (frusemide, thiazides) although effusions may be well tolerated.

d. Immunosuppressive drugs (e.g. prednisolone) *may* help.

In the absence of uraemia, the prognosis may be quite good—recovery may be total.

In the presence of uraemia, treatment is unlikely to succeed.

N.B. The level of urinary protein is *not* a guide to the degree of renal disease and the presence of protein in urine does *not* necessarily indicate renal failure: more commonly it originates from the lower urinary tract.

REFERENCES AND FURTHER READING

Allen T. A. and Jaenke R. S. (1981) Pyelonephritis in the dog. *Compend. Cont. Ed. Pract. Vet.* **7**, 421.

Bovee K. C. (1976) The uremic syndrome. *J. Am. Anim. Hosp. Assoc.* **12**, 189.

Bovee K. C. (1979) Dietary protein and chronic renal failure in dogs. In: Grunsell C. S. G and Hill F. W. G. (ed.) *Veterinary Annual.* Bristol, Wright Scientechnica.

Bush B. M. (1972) A review of the treatment of canine renal disease. *Vet. Rec.* **90**, 669.

Eriksen K. aand Grondalen J. (1984) Familial renal disease in soft-coated wheaten Terriers. *J. Small Anim. Pract.* **25**, 489.

Finco D. R. and Barsanti J. A. (1979) Bacterial pyelonephritis. *Vet. Clin. N. Am.* **9**, (4), 645.

Gourley J. M. and Parker H. R. (1977) Peritoneal dialysis. In: Kirk R. W. (ed.), *Current Veterinary Therapy VI.* Philadelphia, Saunders.

Jackson R. F. (1964) The use of peritoneal dialysis in the treatment of uraemia in dogs. *Vet. Rec.* **76**, 1482.

Jeraj K., Osborne C. A. and Stevens J. B. (1982) Evaluation of renal biopsy in 197 dogs and cats. *J. Am. Vet. Med. Assoc.* **181**, 367.

Kelly D. F., Haywood S. and Bennett A. M. (1984) Copper toxicosis in Bedlington Terriers in the United Kingdom. *J. Small Anim. Pract.* **25**, 293.

McEwan A. D. (1971) The clinical diagnosis of renal disease in the dog. *J. Small Anim. Pract.* **12**, 543.

Mackenzie C. P. and Van den Broek A. (1982) The Fanconi syndrome in a Whippet. *J. Small Anim. Pract.* **23**, 469.

Maddison J. E., Pascoe P. J. and Jansen B. S. (1984) Clinincal evaluation of sodium sulfanilate clearance for the diagnosis of renal disease in dogs. *J. Am. Vet. Med. Assoc.* **185**, 961.

Osborne C. A. (1970) Urologic logic—diagnosis of renal disease. *J. Am. Vet. Med. Assoc.* **157**, 1656.

Osborne C. A. (1974) Dietary restriction in the treatment of primary renal failure: facts and fallacies. *J. Am. Anim. Hosp. Assoc.* **10**, 73.

Osborne C. A. (1974) Percutaneous renal biopsy. In: Kirk R. W. (ed.) *Current Veterinary Therapy V.* Philadelphia, Saunders.

Osborne C. A., Finco D. R. and Low D. G. (1972) *Canine and Feline Urology.* Philadelphia, Saunders.

Osborne C. A., Johnson K. H. and Perman V. (1969) Amyloid nephrotic syndrome in the dog. *J. Am. Vet. Med. Assoc.* **154**, 1545.

Osborne C. A., Low D. G. and Finco D. R. (1969) Reversible versus irreversible renal failure in the dog. *J. Am. Vet. Med. Assoc.* **155**, 2062.

Parker H. R. (1980) Current status of peritoneal dialysis. In: Kirk R. W. (ed.), *Current Veterinary Therapy VII.* Philadelphia, Saunders.

Polzin D. J., Osborne C. A., Hayden D. W. and Stevens J. B. (1983) Effects of modified diet in dogs with chronic renal failure. *J. Am. Vet. Med. Assoc.* **183**, 980.

Steward A. P. and Macdougall D. F. (1984) Familial nephropathy in the cocker spaniel. *J. Small Anim. Pract.* **25**, 15.

Wright N. G., Fisher E. W., Morrison W. I. et al. (1976) Chronic renal failure in dogs: a comparative clinical and morphological study of chronic glomerulonephritis and chronic interstitial nephritis. *Vet. Rec.* **98**, 288.

Chapter 29

Lower Urinary Tract Disorders

A. CONGENITAL LESIONS (Pearson and Gibbs, 1971)

1. Absence of bladder.
2. Ectopic ureter ± ureterocele (common in ♀ > ♂).
3. Immature bladder—fails to distend adequately.
4. Functional disturbance to bladder sphincter.
5. Pervious urachus.

Signs

True incontinence (*see* Chapter 32 for investigation).

B. URINARY INFECTIONS

(Cystitis, prostatitis, urethritis.)
1. Caused by ascending infection.
2. May readily spread from one site to another (occasionally may reflux → pyelonephritis).
3. Occur more readily in females than males.
4. Exacerbated by:
    a. Urinary obstruction.
    b. Urinary retention.
    c. Trauma.

Signs (acute or recurrent)

    a. Frequency of urination with tenesmus.
    b. Small quantities passed.

    c. Haematuria (common).

    d. Incontinence (occasionally).

    (N.B. infections may cause no signs.)

Findings

Often minimal:

    a. Abdominal palpation:

        i. Small, thickened bladder?

        ii. Pain on palpation of the bladder?

    b. Rectal palpation:

        Prostatic pain?

Investigations

    a. Catheterization (direct cystocentesis is better):

        i. Check for absence of obstruction.

        ii. Provides an uncontaminated urine sample.

    b. Urine analysis:

        i. Usually alkaline pH.

        ii. Deposit—usually R.B.C., W.B.C. and bacteria.

        iii. Blood and protein are usually present.

        iv. Normal concentration.

    c. Urine culture and sensitivity:

        Typical agents: *E. coli,* streptococci, staphylococci,
        Pseudomonas, Proteus spp. Klebsiella.

        (significant level of infection if $> 10^5$ organisms/ml.)

    d. Radiology (Chapter 35):

        Pneumocystogram helps to identify structures (prostate,
        calculi etc.) and to exclude other diagnoses.

Treatment

    a. Antibacterial

    —use agents frequently (t.d.s.) and for a prolonged period:

        i. Initially use broad-spectrum agents
        (e.g. trimethoprim combinations or amoxycillin).

        ii. Then according to sensitivity or mean inhibitory tests:
        Ideally—if urine pH is > 7, use erythromycin or
        streptomycin; if urine pH is < 7, use penicillins or
        tetracyclines.

    a. Encourage thirst and fluid intake (add salt to food?):

        i. Add water or gravy to food.

        ii. Provide ready access to water at all times.

    c. Acidify urine (if alkaline): or use ascorbic acid (vitamin C) Chlorethamine (Intervet).

If infections persist—check for:

    a. Other disease (calculi, neoplasia).
    b. Residual urine in bladder/bladder diverticulum/urachus.
    c. Poor client compliance in prolonged antibiotic therapy:
        i. If necessary, use for a long time at a low level.
        ii. Especially if administered after last urination at night.

C. URINARY OBSTRUCTION

1. Calculi:
    a. Phosphate (struvite)—most common—favoured by:
        i. Infection (especially staphylococci and proteus).
        ii. Alkaline urine.
        iii. Bitches>dogs.
    b. Cystine (renal tubule defect—male dogs: heritable?).
    c. Oxalate
    d. Urate—especially with hepatic failure and in Dalmations.

The bladder and urethra are more commonly affected than kidneys and ureters in dogs.

Calculi are most common in Corgis, Dachshunds and Cairns: uncommon in large breeds and working dogs.

2. Prostatic disorders (*see* Chapter 30).
3. Adhesions following trauma or surgery.
4. Neoplasia of the bladder, urethra, prostate or vagina.
5. Pressure of abdominal masses.
6. Retroflexed bladder (perineal hernia).
7. Penile trauma.
8. Idiopathic.

Signs

    a. Tenesmus, pain on urination—persistent or recurrent.
    b. Haematuria (blood in or at the end of urination).
    c. Dripping or dribbling of urine.

Findings

    a. Abdominal palpation:
        i. Firm, enlarged bladder.
        ii. Pain and tenesmus on palpation?
        iii. Calculi are occasionally palpable.

    b. Rectal examination:
        i. Urethral obstruction is occasionally palpable.
        ii. Perineal hernia and retroflexed bladder?

Investigations

    a. Catheterization:
        i. Any obstruction to flow? (Back-flush with saline).
        ii. Is any blood early or late in the flow?
    b. Urine analysis:
        i. Check the pH.
        ii. Deposit—check the type of crystals.
        iii. Blood and protein are often present.
        iv. Presence of bacteria? → urine culture?
  N.B. The presence of crystals in urine is often not significant.
    c. Check renal function—esp. plasma urea and potassium levels.
    d. Radiography (Chapter 35):
        i. Phosphate, oxalate (±cystine) calculi are usually visible in the bladder or urethra on plain films.
        ii. A pneumocystogram is very useful to indicate the position and contents of the bladder and to indicate any stricture.
        iii. Retrograde urethrography may be helpful.
        iv. (Evidence of hydronephrosis *may* be seen.)

Treatment

    a. Sedate or anaesthetise, catheterise and try to flush calculi into bladder with saline.
    b. Institute intravenous fluid therapy.
    c. Surgical relief may be necessary.
    d. Eliminate any infection (*see* p. 171).
    e. Attempt to discourage recurrence or growth of calculi:
        i. Allow frequent opportunities to urinate.
        ii. Provide water at all times and add to food.
        iii. Encourage thirst (*see* p. 171).
        iv. Attempt chemical suppression:
            Phosphates: acidify the urine?
              Ascorbic acid (vitamin C).
              Chlorethamine (Intervet).
              DL-methionine.
              Urease inhibitors? (acetohydroxamic acid 25 mg/kg/day) (Osborne et al., 1981).

Diet:

Cystine and urates: alkalinize:
  With oral sodium bicarbonate?
  Reduce the protein intake?
Oxalates: reduce calcium intake?
Cystines: D-penicillamine (2·5 mg/kg day).
Urates: allopurinol (30 mg/kg body weight/day).

f. Check renal function (hydronephrosis, post-renal uraemia?) and treat if necessary (Chapter 28).

D. URINARY TRACT NEOPLASIA

1. Transitional-cell carcinoma (bladder).
2. Papilloma (bladder).
3. Prostatic carcinoma.
4. Vaginal polyp (leiomyoma) (usually benign).
5. Penis or prepuce.

Signs

a. Haematuria.
b. Dysuria (tenesmus/frequency).
c. Retention of urine.

Findings

a. Visual inspection (penis or vagina).
b. Abdominal palpation: enlarged prostate? thickened bladder?
c. Rectal examination: large irregular prostate?
             irregularities at the bladder neck?

Investigations

a. Catheterization:
   i. Obstruction to flow?
   ii. Blood in the urine?—at what stage?
   iii. Cytology: neoplastic cells?
b. Radiology (Chapter 35):
   i. Pneumocystogram is very helpful.
   ii. Positive contrast or double contrast if in any doubt (especially for bladder and prostate).

Treatment

Usually unsuccessful—involvement of tissues is too great *but* papillomas and vaginal polyps may be removed successfully.

E. LOWER URINARY TRACT TRAUMA

1. Ruptured bladder, urethra or ureters.
2. Haemorrhage or blood clots (kidney, bladder, urethra).
3. Fibrosis or obstruction (*see* p. 172).

Signs of ruptured lower urinary tract

 a. May be those of *acute renal failure* (Chapter 28), a few days
  after an accident.
   i. Anorexia, lethargy, vomiting, halitosis.
   ii. Often some urine is still passed, but reduced in quantity.
 b. Haematuria.
 c. Anuria.

Findings

 a. Rupture—bladder may not be palpable.
 b. Renal haemorrhage—pallor, pain?

Investigations

 a. Ascitic fluid—ammoniacal smell, very high urea content.
 b. Rising plasma urea (if acute renal failure).
 c. Radiology:
   i. Absence of bladder shadow.
   ii. Air in abdomen following pneumocystogram.
   iii. Obstruction? (p. 172).

Treatment

Surgical—if obstruction or rupture, otherwise haemorrhage may resolve
without treatment.

F. MISCELLANEOUS URINARY DISORDERS

1. Haemorrhage cystitis: idiopathic—not common:
 confirmed with an exploratory laparotomy.
2. Emphysematous cystitis:
 occasionally detected radiographically in diabetes mellitus.

REFERENCES AND FURTHER READING

Burnie A. G. and Weaver A. D. (1983) Urinary bladder neoplasia in the dog, a review of
 seventy cases. *J. Small Anim. Pract.* **24,** 129.
Bush B. M. (1976) A review of the aetiology and consequences of urinary tract infections
 in the dog. *Br. Vet. J.* **132,** 632.

Greene R. W. and Scott R. C. (1983) Diseases of the bladder and urethra. In: Ettinger S. J. (ed.), *Textbook of Veterinary Internal Medicine,* 2nd Ed. Philadelphia, Saunders.

Hayes H. M. (1984) Breed associations of canine ectopic ureter: a study of 217 female cases. *J. Small Anim. Pract.* **25,** 501.

Holt P. E. Gibbs C. and Pearson H. (1982) Canine ectopic ureter—a review of twenty-nine cases. *J. Small Anim. Pract.* **23,** 195.

Ling G. V. (1979) Treatment of urinary tract infections. *Vet. Clin. N. Am.* **9**(4), 795.

Osborne C. A. (1980) Genitourinary Disorders. In: Kirk R. W. (ed.), *Current Veterinary Therapy VII.* Philadelphia, Saunders.

Osborne C. A., Abdullahi S., Klausner J. S., Johnston G. R. and Polzin D. J. (1983) Nonsurgical removal of uroliths from the urethra of female dogs. *J. Am. Vet. Med. Assoc.* **182,** 47.

Osborne C. A., Klausner J. S., Krawiec D. R. et al. (1981) Canine struvite urolithiasis: problems and their dissolution. *J. Am. Vet. Med. Assoc.* **179,** 239.

Osborne C. A., Low D. G. and Finco D. R. (1972) *Canine and Feline Urology.* Philadelphia, Saunders.

Owen R. ap R. (1973) *Canine ectopic ureter (I and II) J. Small Anim. Pract.* **14,** 407 and 419.

Pearson H. and Gibbs C. (1971) Urinary tract abnormalities in the dog. *J. Small Anim. Pract.* **12,** 67.

Pechman R. D. (1982) Urinary trauma in dogs and cats: a review. *J. Am. Anim. Hosp. Assoc.* **18,** 33.

Chapter 30

Prostatic Disorders

The prostate gland is a hormone-sensitive organ.
Most disorders are found in ageing dogs.

A. HYPERPLASIA (acinar—favoured by androgens)

Very common in normal ageing dogs.

Signs

Urinary and/or faecal tenesmus, or constipation.
Signs may be minimal. Occasional haemorrhage.

Findings

Symmetrical, painless enlargement—may be intra-abdominal.
Diagnosed by rectal or abdominal examination and radiology.

Treatment (*see* p. 180)

    a. Oestrogens—stilboestrol or oestradiol.
    b. Androgen antagonists (e.g. Tardak; Syntex).
    c. Castration.

B. INFECTION/ABSCESSATION

1. Acute prostatitis—uncommon (usually due to ascending infection)

Signs

Acute and severe pain, stiff gait, arched back, depression, inappetance, malaise (vomiting), unwillingness to defaecate or urinate, dysuria.

Findings

Pyrexia, marked prostatic pain and tension. Abdominal guarding. Leucocytosis and W.B.C. and R.B.C. in urine.

2. Chronic infection

Very common, may often be involved with cystitis.

Signs

    a. Urinary frequency and tenesmus, haemorrhage.
    b. May be pyuria or dribbling of pus±pyrexia.

Findings

    a. Fluctuant swelling of prostate.
    b. W.B.C., R.B.C. and bacteria in urine.

3. Abscessation

May result from:
    a. Oestrogen treatment for benign hyperplasia.
    b. Cystic metaplasia (e.g. Sertoli cell tumour).

Signs

Can cause peritonitis, dysuria, tenesmus, pain, pyuria, haematuria.

Findings

Similar to 1, but usually less severe.

General treatment

Very difficult to clear infections—can try:
    a. Urinary catheter and rectal pressure.
    b. Paracentesis—with a needle at the ischiorectal fossa.
    c. Marsupialization (Hoffer, Dykes and Greiner, 1977).
    d. Antibiotics at high levels and for long periods of time.
    e. Prostatectomy (difficult and unrewarding).

C. NEOPLASIA (adenocarcinoma or sarcoma)—not common.

Signs

May be haematuria and urinary obstruction (and weight loss) and similar signs to those of hyperplasia.
The tumour may not be evident until adjacent spread occurs.

Findings

> a. Irregularly enlarged prostate? Pain?
> b. Sublumbar lymph nodes may be enlarged on radiographs.
> c. Neoplastic cells in urine?

Treatment

Almost impossible in dogs.

D. PROSTATIC HAEMORRHAGE

Recurrent spontaneous haemorrhage (especially with hyperplasia):
Haemorrhage may be after urination or independent of urination.
May respond well to oestrogens.

E. CYSTIC METAPLASIA

Especially with a Sertoli cell testicular tumour or oestrogen therapy.

Signs

May not be evident until very large.

Findings

Fluctuant swelling (soft) with a rectal examination.
Diagosed radiographically.

Treatment

May require drainage or marsupialization and castration.

F. PARAPROSTATIC CYST

1. An occasional finding with radiology.
2. Usually of little significance although dysuria can occur.

GENERAL SIGNS AND MANAGEMENT OF PROSTATIC DISEASE

1. Faecal tenesmus: may be constipation or ribbon-like faeces (A, C, E).
2. Urinary tenesmus or incontinence (may occur with A, B, C, E,).

3. Haematuria: blood after or independent of urination (B, C, D).
4. Pyuria or passage of pus independent of urination (with B, E).
5. Abdominal discomfort (especially B, C).

Investigations

    a. Rectal examination: prostate may be intrapelvic or abdominal. Enlargement may be:
        i. Smooth (hyperplasia or cyst).
        ii. Irregular (neoplasia).
        iii. Firm and painful (prostatitis).
        iv. Soft and fluctuant (cystic metaplasia).
    b. Palpate abdomen—pain? (prostatitis).
    c. Urinary catheterization (with simultaneous rectal exam?) Sample for analysis and bacteriology (blood, pus, other cytology?) (infection or neoplasia?).
    d. Radiology (Chapter 35):
        i. The prostate is normally visible on plain radiographs —if in doubt, carry out pneumocystography.
        ii. Enlargement may be intrapelvic or intra-abdominal.
        iii. Neoplasia is best demonstrated with positive contrast.
        iv. Neoplasia may be invasive—check sublumbar lymph nodes.
    e. Biopsy—especially if no response to treatment. Using a biopsy needle through the ischiorectal fossa (Weaver, 1977) or excising a wedge at exploratory laparotomy.

General treatment for prostatic disease

    a. Oestrogens—if hyperplasia/haemorrhage/(neoplasia):
        i. Oestradiol (Intervet) 0·5–1·0 mg/day s.c. for 5 days or 5–10 mg s.c. weekly.
        ii. Stilboestrol 1–3 mg/day for 5 days (then 0·5 mg three times weekly).
N.B. Excess may cause metaplasia and thrombocytopenia.
    b. Castration or anti-androgens—if hyperplasia or metaplasia Delmadinone 1–3 mg/kg s.c. (Tardak; Syntex).
    c. Antibacterial agents—if infection or abscessation:
        i. Prolonged administration is required (poor penetration).
        ii. Trimethoprim combinations are particularly useful.
    d. Drainage of prostatic abscess or cyst:
        i. With a urinary catheter and rectal pressure.
        ii. By needle.
        iii. By marsupialization (for cysts or abscessation) (Hoffer, Dykes and Greiner, 1977).

REFERENCES AND FURTHER READING

Barsanti J. A. and Finco D. R. (1979) Canine bacterial prostatitis. *Vet. Clin. N. Am.* **9**, (4) 679.

Barsanti J. A. and Finco D. R. (1984) Evaluation of techniques for diagnosis of canine prostatic diseases. *J. Am. Vet. Med. Assoc.* **185**, 198.

Borthwick R. and Mackenzie C. P. (1971) The signs and results of treatment of prostatic disease in dogs. *Vet. Rec.* **89**, 374.

Campbell J. R. and Lawson D. D. (1963) The signs of prostatic disease in the dog. *Vet. Rec.* **74**, 4.

Greiner T. P. and Johnson R. G. (1983) Diseases of the prostate gland. In: Ettinger S. J. (ed.) *Textbook of Veterinary Internal Medicine*, 2nd Ed. Philadelphia, Saunders.

Hoffer R. E., Dykes N. L. and Greiner T. P. (1977) Marsupialization as a treatment for prostatic disease. *J. Am. Anim. Hosp. Assoc.* **13**, 98.

Hornbuckle W. E. and Kleine L. J. (1980) Medical management of prostatic disease. In: Kirk R. W. (ed.) *Current Veterinary Therapy VII*. Philadelphia, Sunders.

Ling G. V., Branam J. E., Ruby A. L. and Johnson D. L. (1983) Canine prostatic fluid: techniques of collection, quantitiative bacterial culture, and interpretation of results. *J. Am. Vet. Med. Assoc.* **183**, 201.

Stone E. A., Thrall D. E. and Barber D. L. (1978) Radiographic interpretation of prostatic disease in the dog. *J. Am. Anim. Hosp. Assoc.* **14**, 115.

Weaver A. D. (1977) Trans-perineal punch biopsy of the canine prostate gland. *J. Small Anim. Pract.* **18**, 573.

Weaver A. D. (1980) Prostatic disease in the dog. In: Grunsell C. S. G. and Hill F. W. G. (ed.), *Veterinary Annual*. Bristol, Wright Scientechnica.

Chapter 31

Differential Diagnosis and Investigation of Haematuria

Blood (and protein) in the urine may arise from any level of the urinary tract.
1. Kidneys:
    a. Trauma.
    b. Neoplasia
    c. Pyelonephritis.
    d. Calculus.
    e. Infarction.
    f. Acute renal failure (toxic or leptospiral).
Produce diffuse haemorrhage—may be only *microscopic* blood.
2. Ureters (uncommon)—calculus.
3. Bladder:
    a. Trauma.
    b. Cystitis:
        i. Bacterial.
        ii. Uroliths (calculi).
        iii. Retention.
        iv. Idiopathic/haemorrhagic.
    c. Neoplasia.
Usually produce diffuse haemorrhage—may be dark in colour.
4. Prostate:
    a. Trauma
    b. Infection.
    c. Neoplasia.
    d. Hyperplasia.
    e. Spontaneous, idiopathic haemorrhage.
There may be haemorrhage independently of urination.

5. Urethra:
   a. Trauma.
   b. Urethritis
      i. Bacterial.
      ii. Calculi.
Usually the haemorrhage is during or at the end of urination.
6. Female genital tract:
   a. Pro-oestrus/abnormal oestrus.
   b. Metritis/pyometra.
   c. Vaginitis/neoplasia.
   d. Parturition/trauma.
7. Penis/prepuce:
   a. Trauma.
   b. Neoplasia.
8. Coagulopathy.
9. (Septicaemia/toxaemia/viraemia.)

Tenesmus is also frequently present if a lower urinary tract disorder is the cause.

INVESTIGATION OF HAEMATURIA

History

   a. Is it a *true* haematuria? (or haemoglobinuria or drugs?)
      (A client may be confused by haematemesis, dysentery or other loss.)
   b. Is the blood:
      i. Diffuse in urine? (bladder or renal disorders).
      ii. At the end of urination? (lower urinary tract).
      iii. Separate from urine? (prostatic disorders).
   c. Persistence/recurrence/frequency.
   d. Tenesmus present? (cystitis, calculi, obstruction).
   e. Oestrus/reproductive history.

Findings

   a. Examine external genitalia: penile or vaginal trauma or neoplasm?
   b. Palpate the abdomen:
      i. Bladder—pain? (tumour/trauma/calculi).
      ii. Kidneys—pain or enlargement? (trauma/tumour/inflammation).
      iii. Other tumour?
   c. Vaginal examination (speculum or digital):
      i. Neoplasia.

      ii. Vaginitis.
     iii. Discharges?
  d. Rectal examination:
      i. Prostatic enlargement or pain? (Chapter 30).
     ii. Urethral calculus or tumour? (Chapter 29).

Investigations

  a. Check for *coagulopathy* (Chapter 42).
  b. *Urinary catheterization*—advantages:
      i. Calculi or obstructions are readily detected.
     ii. Detection of blood:
        In urine.
        Separate from urine?
    iii. Yields a truly cystic urine sample for:
        Analysis (including microscopy on the deposit).
        Culture.
N.B.   i. Direct cystocentesis (using a needle trans-abdominally) gives a pure bladder sample.
     ii. Any haematuria will be associated also with proteinuria.
    iii. Check that R.B.C. are present, not myoglobin or haemoglobin.
  c. Check haematology (anaemia, haemolysis, abnormal platelets?)
  d. *Radiography* (Chapter 35):
      i. Plain films:
        Urinary calculi?
        Renal/prostatic/uterine enlargement?
     ii. Contrast studies:
        Pneumocystogram—useful for identifying:
          Cystic neoplasia or calculi.
          Site and size of prostate.
        Intravenous urography—useful for identifying:
          Upper urinary tract neoplasia or calculi.
        Positive contrast cystography—for identifying:
          Lower urinary tract calculi or neoplasia.
  e. *Exploratory laparotomy*
    Check the bladder, prostate and possible renal biopsy?

FURTHER READING

Meyer D. J. and Senior D. F. (1983) Hematuria and dysuria. In: Ettinger S. J. (ed.) *Textbook of Veterinary Internal Medicine,* 2nd Ed. Philadelphia, Saunders.
Stone E. A., DeNovo R. C. and Rawlings C. A. (1983) Massive hematuria of nontraumatic renal origin in dogs. *J. Am. Vet. Med. Assoc.* **183,** 868.

Chapter 32

Differential Diagnosis and Investigation of Urinary Incontinence

(Involuntary passage of urine)

Bladder control is very complex. It involves sympathetic, parasympathetic and somatic pathways, reflexes and higher CNS centres. Voluntary emptying requires coordination between detrusor muscles, two 'sphincters' and abdominal pressure.

Incontinence is usually caused by one of several mechanisms (Holt, 1983):
1. Raised pressure on the bladder body and/or reduced urethral or bladder neck pressure/resistance.
2. By-passing of the bladder by a urethra.
3. Leakage of urine retained in genitalia between micturitions.

Aetiology

Urinary tract disorders

   a. Congenital malformations
      i. Ectopic ureter or ureterocele.
      ii. Immature bladder.
      iii. Abnormality of the bladder body, neck or urethra.
      iv. Patent urachus.
   b. Spayed bitches (especially large breeds):
      i. 'Hormone imbalance' (shortened bladder neck?)
      ii. Uterine stump adhesions.
   c. Neoplasia—bladder/(urethra)/vagina.
   d. Paradoxical incontinence (due to adhesions/calculi/cystitis).
   e. Bladder neck lesions (calculi/inflammation/trauma).
   f. Displacement of bladder (e.g. by a mass or perineal hernia).
   g. Prostatic disorders (Chapter 30).
   h. Ureterovaginal fistula.

185

Neurological disorders

    a. Prolapsed intervertebral disc.
    b. Skull/spinal/pelvic trauma.
    c. Congenital spinal/CNS lesion.
    d. Neoplastic pressure on nerves.
    e. Detrusor/sphincter incoordination.
       i. Idiopathic.
       ii. Following prolonged distension.

Behavioural and other disorders
(To be differentiated from true incontinence)

Inappropriate urination:
    a. Immaturity.
    b. Poor training.
    c. Senility.
    d. Psychological—excitement/fear/nervousness.
    e. Idiopathic.
    f. Polyuria (nocturia).

INVESTIGATION OF URINARY INCONTINENCE

1. History

    a. Age and sex: young ♀: ectopic ureter? infantile bladder?
                older spayed ♂: hormonal incontinence?
                (especially if spayed young).
    b. Duration of incontinence:
       i. Since birth? (congenital?).
       ii. Recent onset (acquired).
    c. Is it true incontinence? (rather than intermittent wetting):
       i. Wet bed when the animal is lying or moving.
       ii. Constantly soiled coat, smelling of urine.
       iii. Lack of guilt or awareness about urinating in the house.
       iv. Dripping of urine with activity.
    d. Is there polydipsia and *polyuria*? (rather than true
        incontinence).
    e. Ability also to urinate normally?
    f. Ability to defaecate (neurological disorder?)
    g. CNS disease?
       i. Previous trauma?
       ii. Other signs?
    h. History of other surgery?

2. Findings

a. Signs of *CNS dysfunction?*
   i. Conduct a neurological examination.
   ii. Check the perineal reflex.
b. *Observe* urination.
c. *Bladder:*
   i. Full (retention and overflow?)—suggests spinal or peripheral nerve damage.
   ii. Empty (true incontinence).
d. Are the *genitalia* normal? (check vagina in bitches).
e. *Rectal examination* and sphincter tone?
   —prostate and urethra (neoplasia/obstruction?).
f. *Catheterization:*
   i. Obstruction?
   ii. Bladder full or empty?
   iii. Urinary infection?
   iv. Ectopic ureter visible in vagina?

3. Further investigation and management

a. Take samples for:
   i. Plasma urea, glucose.
   ii. Urinalysis (catheterize—obstruction?).
      —to check for polyuric disorders (Chapter 38).
b. If hormonal incontinence is suspected:
   i. Inject 0·5–3·0 mg stilboestrol or oestradiol 1 mg s.c. daily for 3 days.
   ii. Supply 0·5–1 mg tablets daily for 5 days.
      Treatment may need to be repeated from time to time.
      But prolonged oestrogenic therapy should be avoided.
c. Radiology (Chapter 35):
   i. Spine and pelvis (if there are neurological signs).
   ii. Pneumocystogram or double contrast cystography.
   iii. Intravenous urography.
   iv. Vaginourethography.
d. To try to improve bladder tone:
   i. Bethanechol chloride (Myotonine chloride; Glenwood) 5–25 mg t.d.s.
   ii. Distigmine bromide (Ubrebid; Berk) 2·5–5 mg/day.
e. Repeated catheterization to empty a flaccid bladder.
   Or placement of an indwelling catheter to allow drainage; this may permit recovery of bladder tone.
f. Nephrectomy is indicated if a unilateral ectopic ureter is present, or ureterocele or hydronephrosis is detected.
g. Improve sphincter tone?:

    i. Ephedrine 50 mg bid orally (Adams & DiBartola, 1983).

    ii. Phenylpropanolamine?

  h. Surgery to improve bladder function (Holt, 1985)?

N.B. Some forms of bladder dysfunction appear to remain refractory to all logical therapy.

REFERENCES AND FURTHER READING

Adams W. M. and DiBartola S. P. (1983) Radiographic and clinical features of pelvic bladder in the dog. *J. Am. Vet. Med. Assoc.* **182,** 1212.

Bushby P. A. and Hankes G. H. (1980) Sling urethroplasty for the correction of urethral dilatation and urinary incontinence. *J. Am. Anim. Hosp. Assoc.* **16,** 115.

Holt P. E. (1983) Urinary incontinence in the dog. *In Pract.* **5,** 162.

Holt P. E. (1985a) Urinary incontinence in the bitch due to sphincter mechanism incompetence: Prevalence in referred dogs and retrospective analysis of sixty cases. *J. Small Anim. Pract.* **26,** 181.

Holt P. E. (1985b) Urinary incontinence in the bitch due to sphincter mechanism incompetence: surgical treatment. *J. Small Anim. Pract.* **26,** 237.

Holt P. E., Gibbs C. and Latham J. (1984) An evaluation of positive contrast vaginourethography as a diagnostic aid in the bitch. *J. Small Anim. Pract.* **25,** 531.

Michell A. R. (1984) Ins and outs of bladder function. *J. Small Anim. Pract.* **25,** 239.

Oliver J. E. and Bradley W. E. (1974) Treatment of urinary incontinence. In: Kirk R. W. (ed.) *Current Veterinary Therapy V.* Philadelphia, Saunders.

Osborne C. A., Oliver J. E. and Polzin D E. (1980) Non-neurogenic urinary incontinence. In: Kirk R. W. (ed.) *Current Veterinary Therapy VII.* Philadelphia, Saunders.

Pearson H. and Gibbs C. (1971) Urinary tract abnormalities in the dog. *J. Small Anim. Pract.* **12,** 67.

Webbon P. (1982) The radiological investigation of urinary incontinence in the bitch. In: Grunsell C. S. G. and Hill F. W. G. (ed.) *Veterinary Annual.* Bristol, Wright Scientechnica.

Chapter 33

Differential Diagnosis and Investigation of Tenesmus

(A clinical sign: painful straining). The cause can often be determined by careful history-taking and clinical examination.

A. FAECAL TENESMUS (Dyschezia)

1. Constipation—usually *secondary* to:
   a. Pelvic fracture.
   b. Ingestion of bones.
   c. Pain (arthritis or anal lesion).
   d. Prostatic enlargement.
   e. Other disorders (*see below*).
2. Neoplasia—colonic or rectal.
3. Colitis (histiocytic or ulcerative).
4. Enteritis or proctitis.
5. Perineal hernia and rectal sacculation.
6. Megacolon.
7. Rectal or anal stricture.
8. Rectal or anal foreign body.
9. Intussusception or rectal prolapse.
10. Prostatic enlargement.
11. Perianal disorders (usually not much tenesmus):
    a. Fistulae.
    b. Anal sac abscess.
    c. (Adenoma.)

B. URINARY TENESMUS (Dysuria)

1. Bacterial cystitis or urethritis.
2. Cystic or urethral calculi.

3. Trauma or fibrosis involving the lower urinary tract.
4. Neoplasia:
   a. Bladder.
   b. Vagina.
   c. Caudal abdomen.
5. Prostatic disease (hyperplasia/metaplasia/neoplasia/abscess).
6. Bladder displacement:
   a. Perineal hernia.
   b. Ventral rupture.
7. Postoperative or traumatic adhesions (especially uterine stump).
8. Idiopathic.

C. GENITAL TENESMUS

1. Dystocia.
2. Second stage of parturition.

INVESTIGATION OF TENESMUS

History
   a. Frequency of urination and defaecation.
   b. Character of faeces and urine.
   c. Presence of blood in faeces or urine.
   d. Duration and progression of signs.
   e. Posture and position of the tail during tenesmus.
   f. Tenesmus before or after faeces or urine?
   g. Admit for observation if uncertain.

Findings
   a. Anal region:
      i. Perineal hernia.
      ii. Fistulae, abscesses, adenoma.
      iii. Prolapse/intussusception.
   b. Abdomen:
      Palpate (pain?) the bladder, colon, uterus, prostate:
      Enlargement/pain/neoplasia?
   c. Rectal examination:
      i. Discomfort, pain?
      ii. Presence of blood, texture of faeces.
      iii. Character of the anal ring and rectal mucosa.
      iv. Bladder, prostate, urethra, vagina:
         Lesion/obstruction/stricture.
         Displacement/deviation.

     v. Check the pelvis.
  d. Vaginal examination:
     i. Position of the vagina and other structures.
    ii. Abnormal structures? (tumours).
   iii. Cervix and urethra—normal?
  e. Prepuce examination:
    Blood/calculi/neoplasm/trauma?

Investigations

  a. *Catheterization* if urinary tenesmus:
    Ease of passage? (calculi or obstruction?).
    → Uncontaminated sample for analysis.
    → Relief of any obstruction.
    → Contrast radiography.
  b. *Radiography* (Chapter 35)—a valuable aid—may indicate:
     i. Position and contents of the bladder, rectum (uterus).
    ii. Position and size of the prostate.
   iii. Presence of enlarged lymph nodes.
   iv. Presence of abnormal structures (neoplasms).
    v. Presence of calculi.
   vi. Nature of rectal contents (faeces, foreign body?).
  vii. Contrast studies:
    Pneumocystogram (simple and effective).
    Positive contrast or double contrast.
    Intravenous pyelogram/micturating urogram?
    Barium enema/pneumocolography.
  c. *Proctoscopy*—if a faecal problem (*see* Chapter 23).
  d. *Laparotomy* may be required for confirmation of the presence
    of a lesion.

FURTHER READING

Weaver A. D. (1974) Differential diagnosis of tenesmus in the dog. *J. Small Anim. Pract.* **15**, 609.

Chapter 34

Disorders of the
Peritoneal Cavity

A. PERITONEAL EFFUSIONS

A similar range of disorders to those causing pleural effusions (*see* Chapter 3).

1. *Blood:*
     a. Traumatic (especially liver or spleen).
     b. From neoplasm
        (ovarian/hepatic/splenic, especially haemangiosarcoma).
     c. Coagulopathies (*see* Chapter 42).
     d. Perforated peptic ulcer.
     e. (Splenic/gastric torsion).
     N.B. *b* may cause recurrent haemorrhage.

2. *Pus* (uncommon)—peritonitis:
     a. Wounds (especially bites, stakes) penetrating the peritoneum.
     b. Traumatic perforation or organs (especially intestines).
     c. Secondary to rupture of the biliary or urinary tracts.
     d. Secondary to pancreatitis (usually *localized*).
     e. Rupture of the uterus (pyometra or parturition).
     f. Following surgery (swab/infection/suture sinus).
     g. Neoplastic rupture of the alimentary tract.
     h. Foreign body penetration of the alimentary tract.
     Typical agents: streptococci, staphylococci, *E. Coli.*
     Primary agents—Nocardia spp., tuberculosis.

3. *Modified transudate* (common):
     a. Congestive or right-sided cardiac failure.
     b. Hepatic cirrhosis or neoplasia.

      c. Other neoplasms obstructing venous return.

      d. Adhesions following trauma or surgery.

4. *True transudate* (associated with hypoproteinaemias):

      a. Nephrotic syndrome (protein-losing nephropathy).

      b. Protein-losing enteropathy

      c. (Malabsorption or hepatic failure) (uncommonly).

5. *Chyle:*

      a. Traumatic rupture of lymphatics.

      b. Neoplastic rupture or obstruction of lymphatics.

      c. Idiopathic.

6. *Bile*—traumatic rupture of the bile duct or gallbladder
      —often very insidious effusion.

7. *Urine*—ruptured bladder/ureters/urethra.

8. *Neoplastic effusions*—especially carcinomatosis or mesothelioma.

9. *Air/gas:*

      a. Ruptured intestine (trauma/foreign body/tumour).

      b. Abdominal wall wounds.

B. ENLARGEMENT OF OTHER STRUCTURES

1. Uterus (Chapter 37):

      a. Pregnancy.

      b. Pyometra.

      c. Cystic endometrial hyperplasia.

      d. Haemorrhage.

      e. Neoplasia (*rare*).

2. Ovary (Chapter 37):

      a. Cyst.

      b. Neoplasia (may cause generalized neoplasia or ascites).

3. Liver (Chapter 24):

      a. Fatty infiltration.

         i. Hyperadrenocorticalism.

         ii. Diabetes mellitus.

      b. Neoplasia or amyloidosis.

      c. Congestive or right-sided cardiac failure.

4. Spleen (Chapter 26):

      a. Neoplasia.

      b. Splenomegaly.

      c. Torsion.

5. Stomach (Chapter 17):

      a. Overeating.

      b. Gastric dilatation or torsion.

      c. Pyloric obstruction.

6. Intestines: obstruction or constipation (Chapter 21/22).

7. Bladder (Chapter 29):
    a. Atony.
    b. Urethral obstruction.
8. Neoplasms:
    a. Splenic (haemangiosarcoma).
    b. Hepatic.
    c. Mesenteric/renal/pancreatic (carcinomata).
    d. Ovarian.
    e. Testicular (retained).
9. Miscellaneous: obesity, hyperadrenocorticalism, ruptures and hernias cause 'dropped' abdomen.

INVESTIGATION OF ABDOMINAL ENLARGEMENT

History

    a. Speed of onset.
    b. Age (neoplasia?).
    c. Trauma?
    d. Vomiting, polydipsia?

Signs

    a. Shape of the abdomen:
        i. 'Pear-shaped' (ascites).
        ii. 'Dropped' abdomen and skin changes (hyperadreno-corticalism).
        iii. Bloated (gastric dilatation/torsion).
    b. Dyspnoea (? also pleural disease or pressure on the thorax).
    c. Also subcutaneous oedema? (hypoproteinaemia).
    d. Weight loss (especially effusions or neoplasia).

Findings

    a. Tympany (gastric dilatation/torsion).
    b. Fluid wave? (ascites)—very direct.
    c. Palpation:
        i. Unrevealing with ascites or a fat abdomen.
        ii. Hepatic enlargement?
        iii. Bladder size?
        iv. Neoplasia?
    d. Pallor of the mucous membranes if acute haemorrhage.

Investigations

    a. Radiography—look for position of *normal* structures (*see* Chapter 35):
        i. Ascites?

Absence of contrast, loss of outline of normal
structures.
Abdominal distension, ground-glass appearance.
Gas-filled intestines 'floating' in fluid.
  ii. Fluid in a cystic organ (bladder, ovarian cyst/tumour,
uterus)?
  iii. Neoplasm (displacement of intestines and other
organs)?
  iv. Contrast media (Chapter 35):
Use barium to outline the position of the alimentary
tract.
Use air to outline the position of the bladder or colon.
  b. Paracentesis—if fluid is present:
    i. Antisepsis must be maintained.
    ii. With a 19–20 g × 1–in needle:
Enter to one side of the midline, just behind the
umbilicus.
Enter the skin slightly to one side of the site of abdominal
puncture.
    iii. Draw off samples (*see* Chapter 7):
Judge appearance.
Check s.g., proteins (heparin sample bottle).
Check cytology (EDTA bottle).
Bilirubin, urea content?
Culture the fluid if it appears purulent.
    iv. Drain fluid and re-examine the abdomen.
  c. Laboratory findings:
    i. Routine haematology (of limited value):
Leucocytosis and left shift may indicate inflammation or
necrosis.
Anaemia if abdominal haemorrhage?
    ii. Liver enzymes (Chapter 24).
  d. Exploratory laparotomy:
Indicated if a specific lesion is suspected
but it is not a substitute for thorough clinical investigation.

FURTHER READING

Crowe D. T. (1984) Diagnostic abdominal paracentesis techniques: clinical evaluation in
129 dogs and cats *J. Am. Anim. Hosp. Assoc.* **20**, 223.

Chapter 35

Radiographic Findings in Abdominal Disorders

Abdominal radiography has the following special requirements:
1. Abdominal movement must be minimized.
2. Two views (lateral and ventrodorsal) should be taken.
3. Many soft tissues are of similar density, but:
    a. Contrast is enhanced in obesity (e.g. hyperadrenocorticalism).
    b. Contrast is reduced by thinness and by ascites.
    c. Contrast is lacking in young dogs.
    d. Contrast media are often needed to enhance diagnosis.

Structures commonly or normally visible include:
1. Liver—usually cranially to the xiphoid process.
2. *a.* Gastric fundus gas shadow—displaced by the liver or masses.
    b. Pylorus—as a dense or gas-filled structure in left recumbency.
3. Spleen (usually).
4. Bladder (unless empty).
5. Colon, caecum (if faeces or gas are present).
6. Various loops of small intestine.
7. Left (±right) kidney.
Particular attention should be paid to *displacement* of these organs.

Other structures visible if enlarged or diseased, include:
1. Uterus (pyometra, haemometra or pregnancy: enlargement after 3 weeks, foetuses after 6 weeks).
2. Neoplasms (liver/spleen/ovary/kidney/adrenals).
3. Prostate.
4. Lymph nodes.

Prime indications for abdominal radiography include:
1. Acute abdominal disorders (Chapter 20).
2. Persistent vomiting (Chapter 19).
3. Dysuria or haematuria (Chapter 31).
4. Tenesmus (Chapter 33).
5. Identification of a palpable mass.
6. Evaluation of abdominal distension (Chapter 34).
7. Diagnosis of closed pyometra or pregnancy.

Other circumstances where radiography may be helpful include:
1. Hepatic jaundice.
2. Location of a foreign body known to have been ingested.
3. Trauma—to check the bladder, organs for rupture and for free abdominal fluid (e.g. blood).
4. Post-whelping check.
Circumstance where radiography is of little value: chronic diarrhoea.

Significant abnormalities on plain radiographs

1. Signs of effusion (ascites)
    a. Abdominal distension.
    b. Loss of contrast in the abdomen (Difficult to identify normal structures).
    c. General 'ground-glass' opacity, in which
    d. Loops of gas-filled intestine may be visible.
    e. A standing lateral view may demonstrate:
        i. Gas-filled intestines 'floating' in fluid.
        ii. (Occasionally: fluid line.)

2. Homogeneous mass
    a. Bladder?
    b. Hepatic or splenic tumour (cranial abdomen).
    c. Ovarian cyst or renal neoplasm (mid abdomen).
    d. Prostate/prostatic cyst (bladder) (caudal abdomen).
    e. Lipoma or enlarged lymph nodes (lipoma has *decreased* density).

3. Signs of alimentary obstruction
    a. Gross localized dilatation of small intestine—with fluid and gas—especially if:
        i. Wedge-shaped narrowing of the intestine.
        ii. Folded loops of dilated small intestine.
        iii. 'Gravel'—solid material—in dilated loops of small intestines, cranial to the obstruction.
        iv. Gas-capped fluid in loops on a standing lateral view.

　　　b. Delay or obstruction in the passage of contrast material.
　　　c. Dilution of contrast material in dilated intestinal loops.

Aetiology
　　　a. Foreign body/parasitic/neoplastic obstruction.
　　　b. Volvulus/trauma/stricture/adhesions.
　　　c. Intussusception/paralytic ileus.

4. Displacement of abdominal organs
Contrast studies are often required to differentiate between soft tissues of similar densities:
　　　a. To identify the position, size and shape of organs.
　　　b. To identify lesions within an organ (wall/lumen).
　　　c. To assess the function of an organ.

General preparation
If time is available, the following procedures are helpful:
　　　a. Starve the dog of everything except water for 24 hours.
　　　b. Allow dog to *evacuate* colon and bladder.
　　　c. Use an enema and urinary catheterization for (*b*) if needed.
　　　d. Use abdominal compression to improve identification?
　　　e. *Always* examine plain films (2 views) before a contrast study.

1. Barium meal (sedation is not contraindicated)
For upper alimentary studies—*see* Chapter 19:
　　　a. Administer 5 ml/kg body weight of barium (Micropaque; Nicholas Lab) orally (10 ml/kg for double contrast)
　　　b. Radiograph immediately and at ½, 1, 3 and 24 hours.
　　　　　The use of both left and right lateral views may be advantageous for gastric studies.
　　　c. Always re-radiograph a day later to identify delayed passage of barium with intestinal lesions.
　　　d. Double contrast—very good for *pyloric* studies.
　　　　　Air is introduced by stomach tube ½–2 hours after the barium.
　　Normal rates of passage (*very* variable)—contrast material:
　　　a. Enters the duodenum within 20 minutes.
　　　b. Enters the colon within 2 hours.
　　　c. Empties from the stomach within 5 hours.
N.B. A barium meal is of little value in most cases of persistent or recurrent diarrhoea.

Findings
　　　a. Gastric dilatation/foreign body/neoplasia/ulceration.

b. Pyloric spasm or stenosis.

N.B. Considerable variations are found in gastric patterns, and ulceration and neoplasia are not always easily diagnosed.

c. Intestinal obstruction (*see* Chapter 21).

d. Intussusception or linear foreign body (on late films).

2. Barium enema

a. Generally not very helpful (other than for intussusception).

b. The colon must be empty.

c. Light general anaesthesia and atropine are advisable.

d. Procedure:

   i. Administer 10 ml/kg body weight of diluted barium suspension rectally via cuffed tube (Foley catheter or endotracheal tube).

   ii. Radiograph immediately.

   iii. *Stop* administration when contrast reaches the caecum.

   iv. Double contrast gives much more detail of the mucosa:
     Drain out most of the barium.
     Inflate the rectum gently with air or nitrous oxide.

Findings

a. Ilecolic intussusception.

b. Colonic obstruction—neoplasm/stricture/foreign body.

c. Invasive lesion—neoplasia.

d. Masses pressing on the colon.

e. Rectal dilatation or deviation (perineal hernia).

f. (Colonic ulceration?)

3. Pneumocolography

Requires less rigorous preparation? (only sedation is required).
Gently inflate via catheter or tube—with air or nitrous oxide.

Findings: As for (2) *above.*

This is also a simple technique to differentiate colonic from small intestinal gas and to identify abdominal organs in some cases.

4. Pneumocystogram (may be carried out on a conscious animal)

a. Catheterize to remove all urine.

b. Gently introduce (catheter and 3-way tap) 50–200 ml of air.

c. Radiograph immediately—the lateral view is most useful.

Findings

a. Bladder presence/rupture/position.

b. Calculi/neoplasms/prostate position/size (or cyst).

5. Positive cystography

   a. Catheterize and empty the bladder.
   b. Introduce 5 ml/kg of 10–20 per cent iodine solution (Conray; May & Baker. Urografin; Schering).
   c. Radiograph immediately.
   d. *Double contrast*—use only 5–50 ml of positive solution—then introduce 20–100 ml of air.
   e. A micturating urogram can be useful for urethral studies.

Findings

   a. Bladder calculi or neoplasia.
   b. Retrograde ureterograph? (hydroureter).
   c. Prostatic neoplasia or cyst.

6. Intravenous urography—under sedation or general anaesthetic:

   a. Rapid intravenous injection of 1–2 ml/kg body weight iodinated solution (Conray; May & Baker. Hypaque; Winthrop Labs.).
   b. *Immediate* films to record nephrogram.
   c. 3–5 min later to record pyelogram.
   d. 10–30 min for ureters and bladder.
   N.B. The investigation of incontinence may be assisted by the obstruction of the urethra with a catheter or by vaginourethography.

Findings

   a. Renal hypoplasia/infarction/fibrosis.
   b. Renal neoplasia/calculi/cysts.
   c. Hydroureter/pyelonephritis/hydronephrosis.
   d. Ectopic ureter/immature bladder.
   e. Evidence of trauma (ruptured urinary tract).
   f. Whether lesions are unilateral or bilateral.

7. Vagino-urethography (Holt, Gibbs and Latham, 1984)

   a. Fill catheter with dilute contrast (Urografin 150; Schering).
   b. Place catheter:
      ♀ : Foley catheter in vestibule, cuff inflated (close vulva).
      ♂ : urinary catheter → proximal os penis and close prepuce.
   c. Fill bladder—check filling with serial radiographs.
   d. Radiograph in left lateral recumbency.

Findings

   a. Ectopic ureter.
   b. Bladder 'sphincter' dysfunction.
   c. Ureterovaginal fistula or recto-vaginal fistula.

    d. Evidence of uterine stump infection/adhesions.

    e. Urethritis, urethral or vaginal neoplasia.

8. ***Cholecystography***—not much indicated in dogs:

    a. Feed a fatty meal 2 days earlier.

    b. Give no food for 12 hours.

    c. Record a plain film and sedate.

    d. Give oral ipodate (Oragrafin; Schering) (450 mg/kg body weight) 12–16 hours before X-rays *or* i.v. iodipamide (0·5 mg/kg body weight) 1–2 hours before X-rays.

    e. Feed fatty liquid meal (e.g. corn oil) for bile duct study.

    f. Radiograph 30 min later.

Findings

    a. Poor excretion.

    b. Obstruction—neoplasia or calculi (*rare*).

9. ***Portal venography***—to detect portosystemic shunts (Chapter 24)

    a. Exploratory laparotomy
      —to expose the mesenteric or splenic vein.

    b. Introduce 1 ml/kg body weight iodinated solution (Conray; May & Baker).

    c. Radiograph (lateral view of cranial abdomen) immediately.

10. ***Fluoroscopy*** (using an image intensifier)

    a. Valuable in the study of gastric and duodenal functions following the administration of barium.

    b. Valuable in the assessment of excretion urography, especially in identifying an ectopic ureter.

    c. Useful to check function and the extent of penetration of contrast media in colography, cystography and vaginourethography.

    d. Valuable in portal venography.

FURTHER READING

Allan G. S. and Dixon R. T. (1975) Cholecystography in the dog. *J. Am. Vet. Radiol. Soc.* **16,** 98.

Borthwick R. and Robbie B. (1969) Urography in the dog by an intravenous transfusion technique. *J. Small Anim. Pract.* **10,** 465.

Douglas S. W. (1966) Contrast media techniques in radiography. *J. Small Anim. Pract.* **7,** 781.

Douglas S. W. and Williamson H. D. (1980) *Principles of Veterinary Radiography,* 3rd ed. London, Baillière Tindall.

Gibbs C. (1981) Radiological features of liver disorders in dogs and cats. In: Grunsell C. S. G. and Hill F. W. G. (ed.), *Veterinary Annual.* Bristol, Wright Scientechnica.

Gibbs C. and Pearson H. (1973) The radiological diagnosis of gastrointestinal obstruction in the dog. *J. Small Anim. Pract.* **14**, 61.

Holt P. E., Gibbs C. and Latham J. (1984) An evaluation of positive contrast vaginourethography as a diagnostic aid in the bitch. *J. Small Anim. Pract.* **25**, 531.

Johnson G. R., Feeney D. A. and Osborne C. A. (1979) Radiographic findings in urinary tract infection *Vet. Clin. N. Am.* **9**,(4), 749.

Kealy J. K. (1979) *Diagnostic Radiology of the Dog and Cat.* Philadelphia, Saunders.

Kneller S. K. (1976) Radiographic interpretation of the gastric dilatation-volvulus complex in the dog. *J. Am. Anim. Hosp. Assoc.* **12**, 154.

Lee R. and Leowijuk C. (1982) Normal parameters in abdominal radiology of the dog and cat. *J. Small Anim. Pract.* **23**, 251.

Lord P. F., Scott R. C. and Chan K. F. 91974) Intravenous urography for evaluation of renal diseases in small animals. *J. Am. Anim. Hosp. Assoc.* **10**, 139.

O'Brien T. R. (1978) *Radiographic Diagnosis of Abdominal Disorders in the Dog and Cat.* Philadelphia, Saunders.

Thrall D. E. (1977) The abdomen. In: Carlson W. D. (ed.), *Veterinary Radiology.* Philadelphia, Lea & Febiger.

Chapter 36

Endocrine Disorders

Many body functions are influenced by alterations in the *balance* of hormones. Not all upsets involve absolute deficiencies or excesses. The term 'orchestra of hormones' is appropriate: rarely does a single hormone influence a single metabolic process.

Disorders can arise from various disturbances:

a. Failure of releasing factor from hypothalamus.
b. Deficiency of stimulatory hormone.
c. (Excess of inhibiting factor at hypothalamus?)
d. Failure of response by hypothalamus or pituitary to feedback.
e. Inactivation of hormone already released (immune response).
f. Antagonism to hormone by others.
g. Failure of hormone receptors to respond to hormone.
h. Excess hormone or hormone-like substance production by a neoplasm.
i. Administration of excess exogenous hormone (iatrogenic).

A. PITUITARY

1. Panhypopituitarism

Pituitary dwarfism (in growing dogs) (Allan et al., 1978)
Lack of growth hormone especially in German Shepherds.
May also be reduced stimulation of thyroid and adrenal cortex.

Signs

a. Retarded development → early death
   or dwarfing, with normal adult proportions.

203

   b. Soft puppy coat—may → alopecia (esp. in areas of wear).
   c. High-pitched bark, slow learning   ⎫ variable
   d. Infantile genitalia, often docile   ⎬

Findings and investigations
Delayed epiphyseal closure. Poor epiphyseal ossification.
Retained deciduous teeth.
No specific test is readily available, but thyroid and cortisol levels may
be low.

Treatment
Can be treated with growth hormone (bovine origin) but these infantile
dogs may be well accepted by owners.

DIFFERENTIAL DIAGNOSIS OF POOR GROWTH

   a. Pituitary dwarfism.
   b. Congenital hypothyroidism (cretinism).
   c. Congenital deformity—cardiac, hepatic, renal, alimentary.
   d. Chondrodysplasia.
   e. Chronic sepsis or neoplasia (e.g. leukaemia).
   f. Parasitism.
   g. Poor nutrition.

Adult panhypopituitarism
Uncommon—usually a neoplastic disorder.
Can produce:
   a. Hypothyroidism.
   b. Hypoadrenocorticalism.
   c. Hypogonadism—variable).

2. Diabetes insipidus

Should be considered a syndrome rather than a specific disease
—failure of distal renal tubules to concentrate urine.

Aetiology
   a. Failure of ADH (antidiuretic hormone) synthesis or release at
      neurohypophysis (idiopathic, trauma, neoplasia, inflammation)
      ('cranial' diabetes insipidus).
   b. Failure of kidneys to respond to ADH ('nephrogenic' diabetes
      insipidus) (renal fibrosis/necrosis or idiopathic).
   c. Inactivation of ADH (autoimmune).
   d. Antagonism by other hormones, (e.g. glucocorticoids?).

e. Renal adaptation to
ADH release reduced in   } persistent over-hydration
(e.g. in psychogenic polydipsia).

Signs

a. *Severe* polyuria (±nocturia, incontinence).
b. Compensatory severe polydipsia (>200 ml/kg/day).
c. (Dehydration, weight loss?)
d. Usually otherwise *well.*
e. (Occasionally: neurological disturbance if CNS neoplasia.)

Investigation (Chapter 38)

a. Urine s.g. is *low* (1·001–1·006)—always<1·010.
b. Does *not* respond to water deprivation (*see* p.231).
c. Usually responds to ADH (other polyuric disorders may also).
d. Also: urine osmolality is *low*(<250 mosmol/kg)
   plasma osmolality is *high* (<300 mosmol/kg).

Treatment

a. Desmopressin (DDAVP; Ferring):
   i. Injection of 1–4 mg i.m. as required.
   ii. Nose drops (1 drop ever 8 hours).
       Usually effective, but expensive.
b. Thiazide diuretics (paradoxically) may be effective
   (1–2 mg/kg body weight/day).
   Or clorexolone (Nefrolan; May & Baker).
   With partial restriction of sodium intake (*see* p.94).
c. Chlorpropamide (Diabinese; Pfizer) (3 mg/kg body weight/day) may help—
   Potentiates the renal effects of ADH, or stimulates ADH production?
N.B. Diagnose diabetes insipidus with care: treatment is expensive!

Adult acromegaly—due to excess of growth hormone
Aetiology

a. Excess progestogens—in metoestrus (common in middle age)
                       —iatrogenic (especially contraception).
b. Pituitary hyperplasia/neoplasia (uncommon).

Signs

a. Inspiratory noise ± panting.
b. Polydipsia, polyuria, panting.

    c. Thickened skin and skin folds.
    d. Abdominal enlargement.

Findings
    a. Elevated plasma glucose (can be *diabetic*).
    b. Elevated liver enzymes.
    c. Spreading of teeth in gums (in some cases).

Treatment
Withdraw any progestogen therapy, and spay.

B. THYROID

Hormone release is controlled via the hypothalamus/pituitary.
Thyroid hormone:
1. Controls metabolism.
2. Essential for growth and development.
3. Activates growth phase of hair.

1. Congenital hypoplasia (cretinism)
Signs
Dwarfing, with broad skull, short thick legs and kyphosis.

2. Adult Hypothyroidism
Usually young-middle-aged dogs of larger breeds
(German Shepherds, Irish Setters, Retrievers, Boxers, Afghans).

Aetiology
    a. Primary lymphocytic thyroiditis   } 90 per cent of cases.
    b. Idiopathic atrophy or hypoplasia
    c. Secondary TSH (thyroid stimulating hormone) deficiency:
        i. Pituitary tumour   } <10 per cent of cases.
        ii. Idiopathic

    d. Iodine deficiency (rare).
    e. Thyroid tumour (rarely causes dysfunction).
    f. (Dyshormonogenesis).

Signs
Very variable, often vague and insidious in onset:
    a. Usual:
        i. Lethargy, unwillingness to exercise, fatigue.
        ii. Lack of interest, slow movements.
        iii. Intolerance to cold.

    b. Common:
- i. (Bilateral) thinning, dryness of the coat (trunk, back, tail).
- ii. Skin thickening, hyper-pigmentation, comedones, pyoderma, seborrhoea.
- iii. Weight gain without polyphagia (variable).
- iv. Anoestrus/lack of libido.

    c. Occasional:
- i. Constipation, rarely diarrhoea.
- ii. Puffy face, wooden, 'tragic' expression.
- iii. Peripheral neuropathy.
- iv. Congenital cretinism.
- v. Arcus lipoides corneae (corneal lipidosis).

Findings (very variable)

- *a.* Lethargy, little response to handling.
- *b.* Cool, thickened skin, comedones.
- *c.* Slightly subnormal temperature?
- *d.* Pallor of mucous membranes?
- *e.* Testicular atrophy?
- *f.* Usually normal-sized thyroid.
- *g.* Slight bradycardia?—occasionally.
- *h.* Goitre (*rare*).

Investigations

- *a.* *Haematology*—sometimes slight normocytic, normochromic anaemia (PCV approx. 30 per cent).
- *b.* *Chemistry:*
  - i. High cholesterol ($> 7\cdot9$ mmol/l; 300 mg per cent).
  - ii. Thyroid hormones levels (e.g. T4) are reduced.
    But of little value by most unmodified techniques: should be assessed only by radioimmunoassay and not by test kits or most medical laboratories.
    T4 is also reduced with hyperadrenocorticalism and with anti-inflammatory drugs.
- *c.* Uptake of *radio-active substances* is delayed (specialist procedure)
  - i. [131]I.
  - ii. Sodium pertechnetate
    —valuable but difficult to arrange; affected by certain drugs.
    (Normally 11–40 per cent is taken up by 72 hours) (Bush, 1979).

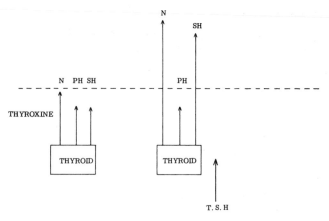

Fig. 11. Interpretation of the TSH stimulation test. Showing responses of T_4 levels before and after TSH stimulation (TSH, thyroid stimulating hormone). - - - - - represents normal level of T_4 before stimulation (often overlaps hypothyroid levels before stimulation). Reproduced from Thoday K. L. (1981) Investigative techniques in small animal clinical dermatology. *Br. Vet. J.* **137**, 133 (*Fig.* 4) by permission.)

    d. *TSH stimulation test* can also be conducted (Bush, 1979); serum samples are collected before and 8 hours after 10 i.u. of TSH i.v.: T4 rises very high in normal animals, rises in *secondary* disease (*see Fig.* 11), with little change in primary hypothyroidism.

    e. *Thyroid biopsy* confirms primary changes.

Treatment

    a. 1-Thyroxine (Eltroxin; Glaxo). Start with 0·02 mg/kg/day in divided doses.

Increase by 0·05 mg weekly, if necessary.

Stop if signs of hyperthyroidism appear.

Care in the presence of cardiac disease.

    b. Thyroid extract is not now indicated (usually an unrefined and poorly stabilized product).

Usual signs of response: increased activity in 7–10 days; hair growth in 1–3 months.

3. Hyperthyroidism

    a. Uncommon—usually due to thyroid tumour.
    b. Iatrogenic—excessive treatment.

Signs

    a. Weight loss with polyphagia.
    b. Heat intolerance, panting.
    c. Nervousness, restlessness.
    d. Polydipsia and polyuria.
    e. Diarrhoea, bulky faeces.

Findings

    a. Cardiomegaly, tachycardia, tachydysrhythmias.
    b. Usually goitre.

Treatment (for primary disease)

    a. Surgical removal of tumour.
    b. Propylthiouracil? (10 mg/kg b.d.)
    c. Withdraw hypothyroid treatment if iatrogenic in origin.
    d. β blockade if tachydysrhythmia (Chapter 11).

4. Neoplasia

Adenoma (benign)—may be few signs.
Carcinoma (especially ageing Boxers)—usually malignant.

Signs

Usually those of adjacent *pressure:*
    a. Regurgitation.
    b. Dyspnoea—with noise.
    c. Oedema of head tissues.
    d. Dysphonia (loss of voice).
    e. (Occasionally: hyperthyroidism or hypothyroidism.)

Findings

    a. Goitre.
    b. Confirmed by biopsy.

Treatment

Usually malignant and resection is difficult or impossible.

5. Hypercalcitonism

(Calcitonin antagonizes parathyroid hormone: inhibits resorption of calcium from bone.)

Has been implicated as a factor in:
- a. Osteochondrosis dissecans.
- b. Hip dysplasia.
- c. Hypertrophic osteodystrophy.
- d. 'Wobbler' syndrome in giant breeds.

(Possibly induced by excessive dietary calcium, vitamin D and protein in fast-growing large breeds of dog.)

C. PARATHYROID

1. Hypoparathyroidism—uncommon

- a. (Accidental removal with thyroid at surgery.)
- b. Idiopathic or lymphocytic parathyroiditis, esp. small dogs?
- c. Neoplasia.

(Lactation tetany ('eclampsia') is effectively a similar disorder due to insufficiently rapid mobilization of calcium.)

Signs

Those of *hypocalcaemia:*
Restlessness, nervousness, hyperexcitability, hyperaesthesia, ataxia, weakness, tremor of individual muscle groups,
hyperventilation, cramp → convulsions (tetany), seizures.

Findings

- a. There may be tachypnoea, tachycardia, pyrexia (as a result of excitability) but bradycardia is likely in later stages.
- b. Low plasma calcium level (<7 mg per cent) (<2 mmol/l). Elevated plasma phosphorus level.
- c. (Confirmed by biopsy).

Treatment

- a. Calcium gluconate 10 per cent *slowly* intravenously (10–20 ml).
- b. High calcium/low phosphorus diet.
- c. Calcium lactate supplementation (0·3 g/kg body weight/ day).
- d. Vitamin D$_3$ (50 000 i.u. initially then 100 i.u. kg/day).
- e. Re-check calcium.

Similar signs can be seen with other causes of hypocalcaemia:
- a. Chronic renal failure.
- b. Diarrhoea/malabsorption.
- c. (Pancreatitis).

2. Hyperparathyroidism

Aetiology

    a. Primary—neoplasia or hyperplasia (uncommon).
    b. Secondary:
        i. Renal hyperparathyroidism.
        ii. Nutritional hyperparathyroidism:
            Low dietary calcium   } especially meat
            High dietary phosphorus
    c. Pseudohyperparathyroidism: secretion of similar hormone
        from:
        i. Lymphosarcoma.
        ii. Carcinomata.
        iii. Multiple myeloma.
        iv. (Apocrine anal sac adenocarcinoma-rare).

Signs

Very variable:
    a. Polydipsia, polyuria, weight loss, exercise intolerance.
    b. Anorexia, depression, gut atony   } (primary, and pseudo disease
    c. Muscle weakness, vomiting   } —with hypercalcaemia)
    d. Skeletal pain (variable), lameness
    e. Reluctance to stand or walk   (secondary disease)

Findings

    a. Bradycardia, dysrhythmias?
    b. ?Dehydration, secondary renal failure } primary disease
    c. Lack of skeletal density (X-ray),
        especially periodontal   secondary
    d. Pathological fractures (painful)
        flexible bones   disease
    e. ECG : prolonged P-Q, shortened Q-T intervals.

Investigation—a complicated disease syndrome

Basic principles:

	Primary	Secondary	Pseudo-
Plasma calcium	high	(low)	high
Plasma phosphorus	low	(high)	low
Alkaline phosphatase	normal to high	raised	normal to high
Biopsy	neoplasia	hypoplasia	atrophy

(Normal plasma calcium: 9·5–11·5 mg per cent (2–3 mmol/l).
Levels of PTH *can* be measured by radioimmunoassay? (Feldman and Krutzik, 1981).

Differential diagnosis of hypercalcaemia
    a. Primary hyperparathyroidism.
    b. Pseudohyperparathyroidism (especially neoplasia).
    c. Hypervitaminosis D.
    d. Malignant bone metastases or osteomyelitis.
    e. Hypoadrenocorticalism.

Treatment
    a. Primary hyperparathyroidism:
       Surgery—with great care to remove only part of the gland?
    b. Hypercalcaemia: intravenous saline, glucocorticoids and frusemide.
    c. Secondary hyperparathyroidism:
       i. Calcium supplementation.
       ii. Oral aluminium hydroxide gel (Mucaine; Wyeth).
       iii. *Rest* and analgesics?
    d. Treatment for renal failure if present (Chapter 28).

Differential diagnosis of generalized loss of skeletal density
    a. Nutritional secondary hyperparathyroidism.
    b. Renal secondary hyperparathyroidism.
    c. Hyperadrenocorticalism.
    d. Rickets (*rare*).

D. ADRENAL

1. Hyperadrenocorticalism (Cushing's syndrome)

A *common* disease syndrome mainly resulting from:
    a. Excess *glucocorticoid* production by the adrenal cortex—due to:
       i. Adrenocortical hyperplasia—secondary to: *either* idiopathic excess ACTH production—(negative feed-back failure?) *or* pituitary neoplasia.
       ii. Adrenocortical neoplasia (usually unilateral).
    b. (Prolonged glucocorticoid therapy.)
Seen in middle-aged or ageing dogs, especially Miniature Poodles, Terriers and Dachshunds

Signs (insidious onset)—variable
    a. Polydipsia and polyuria—about three times the normal water intake.
    b. Polyphagia.
    c. Lethargy, exercise intolerance, muscle weakness.

    d. Weight loss, especially peripheral and temporal muscle atrophy.
    e. Dropped abdomen—due to:
        i. Muscular weakness.
        ii. Inelastic tissues.
        iii. Fat deposition in abdomen and liver.
    f. Thinning of coat, especially flanks, ventral surfaces and thighs → light colour and fine texture.
    g. Anoestrus (and enlarged clitoris?).

Findings

The skin is:
    a. Thinned—blood vessels may be visible under abdominal skin.
    b. 'Lazy'—inelastic and *soft.*
    c. May be melanosis, comedones or calcinosis cutis.
Testicular atrophy may be found. Hepatomegaly is common.
Corneal lipidosis, purpureal haemorrhages may occur.

Investigations

Not simple.
Clinical signs are important.
    a. Haematology:
        i. Slight leucocytosis (neutrophilia).
        ii. Eosinopenia (<200 cells/c mm).
        iii. Usually lymphopenia (<1500 cells/c mm).
    b. Urine is usually poorly concentrated (e.g. $<1 \cdot 012$) but can be concentrated with water deprivation test (Chapter 38). Urinary infection is often found.
    c. Biochemistry:
        i. Liver enzyme (GPT, alkaline phosphatase) raised.
        ii. Cholesterol is raised (>300 mg per cent) ($>7 \cdot 9$ mmol/l).
        iii. Glucose may be elevated (100–120 mg per cent) (6–7 mmol/l).
        iv. Occasionally diabetic.
    d. Radiography:
        i. Hepatomegaly and possible osteoporosis.
        ii. Bronchial ⎫
                    ⎬ calcification may be found.
        iii. Soft tissue ⎭

Confirmation (not relevant in iatrogenic disease)

    a. Plasma cortisol levels are usually elevated
        but normal and abnormal levels overlap.
        Results also vary according to individual laboratory assay.
    Other tests may therefore be conducted:

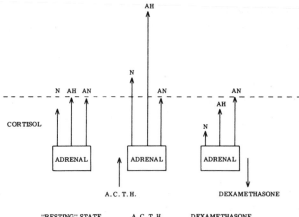

Fig. 12. Interpretation of the ACTH stimulation and dexamethasone suppression tests for hyperadrenocorticalism. Showing responses of plasma cortisol levels before and after tests. (ACTH, adrenocorticotrophic hormone). - - - - - represents an elevated level of cortisol (often overlapped by normal levels at 'rest'—before stimulation). (Reproduced from Thoday K. L. (1981) Investigative techniques in small animal clinical dermatology. *Br. Vet. J.* **137**, 133 (*Fig.* 5) by permission.)

    b. ACTH stimulation test:
       i. Starve the dog.
      ii. Take a morning plasma sample prior to stimulation.
     iii. Inject ACTH analogue:
          10–20 i.u. of Synacthen (Ciba) i.m.
     iv. Re-sample after 2 hours.
Results may indicate the cause (*Fig.* 12)
    c. Dexamethasone suppression test:
       i. Starve the dog.
      ii. Take morning plasma sample prior to suppression.
     iii. Dose orally with dexamethasone (0·1 mg/kg)
     iv. Re-sample 8 hours later.
Results may indicate the cause (*Fig.* 12).
    d. Other tests can also be employed—e.g.:
       Plasma ACTH levels by radioimmunoassay, but gives an overlap with normals.
       (Raised with pituitary form, depressed with adrenal neoplasia)

Differential diagnosis

    a. Other polydipsic disorders, especially diabetes mellitus or insipidus.

    b. Other causes of non-pruritic hormonal alopecia:
        i. Testicular neoplasia or hypoandrogenism.
        ii. Hypothyroidism
        iii. Ovarian imbalance (Chapter 37).

    c. Other cause of abdominal distension (Chapter 34).

Diagnosis and treatment are expensive.

Treatment

If uncertain of the diagnosis, wait and repeat tests after 3 months?

    a. Bilateral adrenalectomy—effective, but postoperative crises due to lack of mineralocorticoids must be mastered.

    b. Unilateral adrenalectomy for tumour? But may be metastases.

    c. Hypophysectomy
      —complicated and drastic but effective (Lubberink, 1980).

    d. Adrenocorticolytic drug *o,p′*DDD (mitotane, Lysodren; Bristol Myers) 50 mg/kg body weight/day until the thirst returns to normal (7–14 days, usually) then a maintenance dose of 50 mg/kg weekly in divided doses (may need adjustment).

N.B. There may be a poor response in the presence of a tumour. Treatment must be *stopped* if severe vomiting, diarrhoea, anorexia or depression occur or when thirst falls markedly. Monitoring of the eosinophil count can be a good guide. For treatment of Lysodren overdosage, *see* hypoadrenocorticalism.

2. Adrenocortical insufficiency (Addison's Disease)

—hypoadrenocorticalism
Uncommon, but it may often be unrecognized.
May result from:

    a. Atrophy of adrenal cortex (? autoimmune) (in young bitches).

    b. Over-treatment of hyperadrenocorticalism with *o,p′*DDD

    c. Sudden withdrawal of corticosteroids after prolonged therapy.

    d. Infiltration of the adrenal cortex by haemorrhage, neoplasm, amyloid or sepsis of the adrenal cortex.

    e. Hypothalamic/pituitary disease reducing ACTH release.

Effect

    a. Mineralocorticoid insufficiency, causing sodium loss, potassium retention and hypovolaemia through failure of renal regulation.

    b. Glucocorticoid deficiency (especially *b* and *c above*).

Signs

    a. Acute: vomiting with anorexia, weakness and collapse. Occurring as 'shock' or failure to recover from anaesthesia, trauma, 'stress' or an alimentary upset.
    or sudden death.

    b. Chronic: a *vague* disorder —signs vary, but may progress: Lethargy, depression, inappetance, weakness, alimentary upsets, weight loss, sometimes polydipsia.

Findings and investigations

    a. Weak pulse, dehydration, poor capillary refill, abdominal pain?

    b. Hypovolaemia, bradycardia (microcardia on radiographs).

    c. Sodium : potassium ratio is usually *low* ($<27 : 1$) (plasma potassium $>5\cdot5$ mEq/l, sodium <135 mEq/l).

    d. Mild (pre-renal) uraemia, with concentrated urine.

    e. Haemoconcentration, sometimes, eosinophilia (mild anaemia).

    f. Hypercalcaemia and hypoglycaemia in some cases.

    g. ECG changes (when K + high):
       i. Bradycardia.
       ii. Elevation and spiking of T waves.
       iii. Suppression of P waves and increased P-Q and QRS intervals.

    h. Low cortisol levels—little affected by ACTH stimulation (p.214).

    i. ACTH level high in atrophy/degeneration, low in pituitary or iatrogenic disease (if it can be measured).

Treatment

    a. Acute failure requires rapid therapy for hypovolaemic shock:
       i. Saline ($0\cdot9$ per cent) followed by glucose (5 per cent) i.v.
       ii. Glucocorticoids (prednisolone, betamethasone i.v.)
       iii. Mineralocorticoid (deoxycortone—Percorten; Ciba) (1—5 mg i.m.) (or use hydrocortisone $\rightarrow$ both effects). And *check* for:
       urinary output, ECG changes and a fall in K+ and urea.

    b. Chronic failure and further therapy:
- i. Fludrocortisone acetate (Florinef; Squibb) orally (0·1–0·5 mg daily). Adjust, according to plasma K+.
- ii. Add table salt to food daily.
- iii. Allow unlimited access to water.
- iv. Give glucocorticoids initially and at times of stress.
- v. Check plasma sodium and potassium regularly.

It may be possible to withdraw therapy after some weeks.

3. Other adrenal disorders

    a. Oestrogen or androgen production in adrenals can lead to feminization or hypersexuality (especially with neoplasia).
    b. In neutered animals, sexual behaviour may be maintained.
    c. Phaeochromocytomas (*rare*); medulla tumours secrete adrenaline or noradrenaline.

    Findings with phaeochromocytomas are variable: excitability, anxiety, whining, trembling, weakness, tachypnoea, tachycardia, hypertension, slow capillary refill, polydipsia.
(an abdominal tumour may be demonstrated).
Elevated catecholamines can be measured

    Treatment: The neoplasm (usually right-sided) can be removed.

E. PANCREATIC ENDOCRINE DISORDERS

1. Diabetes mellitus

Should be considered a *syndrome* rather than a specific disease.
Absolute/*relative* deficiency of insulin → glucose intolerance.

Aetiology

Often uncertain. It includes:
    a. Reduced production or release of insulin (islet cell degeneration or exhaustion).
    b. Inactivation of insulin or islet cells (immune response).
    c. Antagonism to insulin by other hormones (glucocorticoids, progestogens, growth hormone, adrenaline, thyroid hormone).
    d. Decreased receptor affinity for insulin.
May be unmasked by stress/infection/oestrus.

e. Occasionally *may* be associated with: pancreatic exocrine insufficiency; hyperadrenocorticalism; phaeochromocytoma.

Effect
a. Lack of tissue access to glucose for energy and storage.
b. Tissue *catabolism* and lack of utilization of mobilized fats. This causes:
   i. Hyperglycaemia, osmotic diuresis.
   ii. Ketosis, toxaemia.
   iii. Mobilization of fats and deposition in the liver.

Incidence
a. Quite common—1 : 1000 dogs?
b. Predisposition in certain, mainly small, breeds: Dachshund, Poodle, Samoyed, Spaniel, Terriers.
c. Sex: entire bitches affected more than dogs (approximately 3 : 1)
   (especially common at *metoestrus*—increased growth hormone).
d. Age: 5–11 years at diagnosis (7 years peak).

Signs
Develop over a few weeks:
a. Usually: polydipsia, polyuria, polyphagia, weight loss; the animal is alert.
b. Sometimes: skin disorders (dull coat, seborrhoea, pyoderma), gastrointestinal upsets.
   May be presented with decompensated *ketoacidosis* (uncommon): depression, weakness, tachypnoea, dehydration, vomiting and eventually, coma.

Findings
Variable—various secondary effects:
Lens cataracts, hepatomegaly, urinary tract infections, renal damage.

Investigations
a. Persistent glycosuria, therefore high urine s.g. ($>1\cdot040$).
b. Usually persistent hyperglycaemia (> 150 mg per cent, $8\cdot3$ mmol/l).
c. Other effects according to severity:
   i. Ketones in blood and urine.
   ii. Impaired renal function, often urinary infection.
   iii. Raised liver enzyme and cholesterol levels.
   iv. Leucocytosis.
   v. Lipaemia is common.

Oral Glucose Tolerance Test

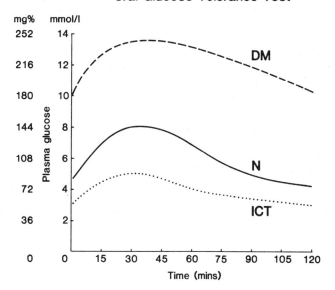

Fig. 13. Interpretation of the oral glucose tolerance test. N, typical curve for normal dogs; DM, typical curve in diabetes mellitus; ICT, typical curve with islet cell tumour.

    d. If in doubt, conduct a *glucose tolerance test:*
     i. Starve the dog for 24 hours.
     ii. Pre-sample for glucose.
     iii. Give 40 per cent glucose (0·r g/kg body weight) i.v. *or* 20 per cent glucose (2 g/kg body weight) orally.
     iv. Sample for glucose at 15–30–60–90–120 min (*see Fig.* 13).

Differential diagnosis of hyperglycaemia
    a. Diabetes mellitus.
    b. Hyperadrenocorticalism.
    c. Pancreatitis.
    d. Acromegaly (adult hyperpituitarism).
    e. Post-prandial or intravenous dextrose.
    f. Stress.
    g. Hepatic failure.
    h. Phaeochromocytoma.
N.B. Additional causes of glycosuria include:
renal failure, Fanconi syndrome, convulsions.

Treatment

This requires a good liaison and discussion with the client: if there is doubt that the client can cope, then treatment may not be worthwhile.

  a. Daily insulin is required.
     (Oral hypoglycaemics or diet adjustment rarely sufficient.)
     Must be maintained even if the client is not available.
  b. Regularity is essential in:
     i. Food intake and diet—usual to feed at least twice daily.
     ii. Time of injection (usually in mornings or twice daily).
     iii. Exercise—keep maintained (little and often?)
     iv. Body weight (unless obese).
  c. Regular urine or blood testing will be necessary (at least once daily at first) until well stabilized, but with experience a client may judge the insulin requirement from the dog's thirst.
  d. Entire bitches should be spayed when stabilized.
  e. Hypoglycaemia is the most likely *crisis*
     —corrected with oral glucose syrup or sugar (*not* insulin).
  f. Diet: unnecessary to alter to low carbohydrates except to reduce obesity. There is merit in feeding high fibre (e.g. bran).
  g. *Ketoacidosis* requires aggressive and intensive therapy:
     i. Intravenous fluids: 50 ml/kg body weight normal saline ±bicarbonate (2mEq/kg body weight)? with care.
     ii. Soluble insulin i.v.: 1 i.u./kg in drip, then i.m.
     iii. Give oral potassium supplementation for a few days.
     iv. Maintain as other diabetics when no longer depressed and anorexic—*monitor* blood glucose and ketones.
  h. Types of *insulin* for maintenance—usually given in the morning or in divided doses (e.g. NPH). The duration is very variable:

	Duration	Peak
Protamine zinc (PZI)	24–36 h	14–20 h
Isophane insulin (NPH)	18–24 h	8–12 h
Zinc lente	18–28 h	10–12 h
Porcine insulin zinc suspension (IZS-P) b.d.	14–16 h	6 h

Stabilization—notes:

  a. The dosage should be built up slowly and blood glucose monitored daily or 4-hourly if unstable in the early stages.
  b. Aim to achieve and maintain:
     a normal blood glucose at the time of peak insulin level.
     or minimal trace of glycosuria in pre-dosage morning sample.
  c. If the dog refuses food, is unwell or requires surgery, glucose may be administered *ad lib,* with two-thirds normal insulin.

    d. If stabilization problems occur, or insulin requirement rises:
       i. Check the client's comprehension and compliance.
      ii. Check the blood glucose 4-hourly.
     iii. Try another form of insulin—e.g. IZS-P or divide →
          b.i.d.
     iv. Consider spaying an entire bitch.
      v. Check for other endocrine diseases causing
         hyperglycaemia.
     vi. Use a fibre-rich diet and divide to feed b.i.d or t.i.d.
Diabetics tend to be prone to further complications
(e.g. skin disorders, gastrointestinal disturbances, urinary infections).

2. Islet cell tumour

    a. Not common, but probably unrecognized in many cases.
    b. Found in ageing dogs, especially Boxers.
    c. Indiscriminate insulin production produces profound hypo-
       glycaemia. (Glucagon-secreting tumours may be found on rare
       occasions.)

Signs

    a. Episodes of trembling and weakness (with disorientation,
       depression, yawning).
    b. Symptoms become more marked over some days or weeks:
       confusion, incoordination, ataxia, apparent blindness, muscle
       twitching.
    c. Seizures or coma may develop.
    d. May be relieved by feeding in some cases.

Findings
Minimal

Investigations

    a. Persistently low blood glucose (<60 mg per cent; 3·4 mmol/l)
       except immediately after feeding?
    b. Elevated insulin levels (>50 µU/ml).
    c. Glucose tolerance test (0·5 g/kg i.v.) gives variable results:
       i. Fairly flat curve.
  or
      ii. Rapid rise and rebound depression (*Fig.* 13).
    d. Insulin: glucose ratio is *high* (> 50 : 1).
       Normal insulin (in µU/ml) : glucose (mg per cent)
       = < 30 : 1.

    e. If the result of *d* is equivocal, assess the Amended Insulin-Glucose Ratio:

$$\frac{\text{insulin (U/ml} \times 100)}{\text{glucose (mg\%)} - 30}$$ —the result in normal dogs is < 30.

    f. If still in doubt, other provocative tests can be tried (e.g. Glucagon Tolerance Test—Johnson, 1977).

Differential Diagnosis

    a. Other causes of seizures:
        i. Encephalitis, hypocalcaemia.
        ii. Epilepsy, poisoning (lead?).
        iii. Hepatic failure, cardiac insufficiency.
        iv. CNS neoplasia.
    b. Other causes of *hypoglycaemia* (all rarer than islet cell tumour):
        i. Functional insufficiency (neonatal, sporting dogs?).
        ii. Other neoplasms (hepatic, other carcinomata).
        iii. Endocrine upsets (hypoadrenocorticalism).
        iv. Glycogen storage diseases, hepatic failure.
    c. Other causes of collapse (Chapter 10).

Treatment

    a. Surgery (with intravenous glucose drip) and *care*:
yhe tumour (often very small and difficult to find) may be resected, but metastases to the liver occur very early. The tumour is most often found in the duodenal limb. Metastases may take months to exert their effects after resection of the primary lesion.
    b. Possibility of the use of diabetogenic agents such as diazoxide (Eudemine) (10 mg/kg/b.i.d.) or to effect?
    c. Other insulin antagonists may be tried: glucocorticoids, propranolol, hydrochlorothiazide.
    d. Feed frequent small meals.

REFERENCES AND FURTHER READING

Allan G. S., Huxtable C. R. R., Howlett C. R. et al. (1978) Pituitary dwarfism in German Shepherd dogs. *J. Small Anim. Pract.* **19**, 711.

Austrad R. and Bjerkas E. (1976) Eclampsia in the bitch. *J. Small Anim. Pract.* **17**, 793.

Belshaw B. E. and Rijnberk A. (1979) Radioimmunoassay of plasma T_4 and T_3 in the diagnosis of primary hypothyroidism in dogs. *J. Am. Anim. Hosp. Assoc.* **15**, 17.

Belshaw B. E. and Rijnberk A. (1980) Hypothyroidism. In: Kirk R. W. (ed.), *Current Veterinary Therapy* VII. Philadelphia, Saunders.

Bush B. M. (1984) Endocrine system. In: Chandler E. A., Sutton J. B. and Thompson D. J. (eds.) *Canine Medicine and Therapeutics*, 2nd Ed. Oxford, Blackwell.

Caywood D. D. and Wilson J. W. (1980) Functional islet cell adenocarcinoma in the dog. In: Kirk R. W. (ed.), *Current Veterinary Therapy* VII. Philadelphia, Saunders.

Chastain C. B. and Nichols C. E. (1981) Low-dose intramuscular insulin therapy for diabetic ketoacidosis in dogs. *J. Am. Vet. Med. Assoc.* **178**, 561.

Church D. B. (1981) The blood glucose response to three prolonged duration insulins in canine diabetes mellitus. *J. Small Anim. Pract.* **22**, 301.

Church D. B. (1982) Canine diabetes emllitus: some therapeutic considerations. In: Grunsell C. S. G. and Hill F. W. G. (ed.), *Veterinary Annual*. Bristol, Wright Scientechnica.

Doxey D. L., Milne E. M. and Mackenzie C. P. (1985) Canine diabetes mellitus: a retrospective survey. J. Small Anim. Pract. **26**, 255.

Eigenmann J. E. (1984) Acromegaly in the dog. *Vet. Clin. N. Am.* **14**, 827.

Eigenmann J. E. and Peterson M. E. (1984) Diabetes mellitus associated with other endocrine disorders. *Vet. Clin. N. Am.* **14**, 837.

Feldman E. C. (1980) Diabetes mellitus. In: Kirk R. W. (ed.), *Current Veterinary Therapy* VII. Philadelphia, Saunders.

Feldman E. C. (1983) Comparison of ACTH response and dexamethasone suppression tests in canine hyperadrenocorticism. *J. Am. Vet. Med. Assoc.* **182**, 506.

Feldman E. C. and Krutzik S. (1981) Case reports of parathyroid levels in spontaneous canine parathyroid disorders. *J. Am. Anim. Hosp. Assoc.* **17**, 393.

Feldman E. C. and Peterson M. E. (1984) Hypoadrenocorticism. *Vet. Clin. N. Am.* **14**, 751.

Greene C. E., Wong P. L. and Finco D. R. (1979) Diagnosis and treatment of diabetes insipidus in two dogs using two synthetic analogs of antidiuretic hormone. *J. Am. Anim. Hosp. Assoc.* **15**, 371.

Hill F. W. G. (1979) Adrenocortical insufficiency in the dog. In: Grunsell C. S. G. and Hill F. W. G. (ed.), *Veterinary Annual*. Bristol, Wright Scientechnica.

Johnson R. K. (1977) Insulinoma in the dog. *Vet. Clin. N. Am.* **7**, 629.

Jones D. E. and Joshua J. O. (1982) *Reproductive Clinical Problems in the Dog*. Bristol, Wright PSG.

Kruth S. A., Feldman E. C. and Kennedy P. C. (1982) Insulin-secreting islet cell tumors: establishing a diagnosis and the clinical course for 25 dogs. *J. Am. Vet. Med. Assoc.* **181**, 54.

Lage A. L. (1973) Nephrogenic diabetes insipidus in a dog. *J. Am. Vet. Med. Assoc.* **163**, 251.

Leifer C. E., Peterson M. E., Matus R. E. and Patnaik A. K. (1985) Hypoglycemia associated with nonislet cell tumor in 13 dogs. *J. Am. Vet. Med. Assoc.* **186**, 53.

Ling G. V., Stabenfeldt G. H., Corner K. M. et al. (1979) Hyperadrenocorticism: pretreatment clinical and laboratory evaluation of 117 cases. *J. Am. Vet. Med. Assoc.* **174**, 1211.

Lubberink A. A. M. E. (1980) Therapy for spontaneous hyperadrenocorticism. In: Kirk R. W. (ed.), *Current Veterinary Therapy* VII. Philadelphia, Saunders.

Mattheeuws D., Rottiers R., DeRijcke J. et al. (1976) Hyperinsulinism in the dog due to pancreatic islet cell tumour: a report on three cases. *J. Small Anim. Pract.* **17**, 313.

Muller G. H., Kirk R. W. and Scott D. W. (1983) *Small Animal Dermatology*. 2nd Ed. Philadelphia, Saunders.

Nelson R. W. and Feldman E. C. (1983) Complications of insulin therapy in diabetes mellitus. *J. Am. Vet. Med. Assoc.* **182**, 1321.

Osborne C. A. and Stevens J. B. 91973) Pseudohyperparathyroidism in the dog. *J. Am. Vet. Med. Assoc.* **162**, 125.

Osborne C. A., Low D. G. and Finco D. (1972) *Canine and Feline Urology.* Philadelphia, Saunders.

Parker A. J., O'Brien D. and Musselman E. E. (1981) Diazoxide treatment of metastatic insulinoma in a dog. *J. Am. Anim. Hosp. Assoc.* **17**, 315.

Peterson M. E. (1982) Treatment of canine and feline hypoparathyroidism. *J. Am. Vet. Med. Assoc.* **181**, 1434.

Peterson M. E. (1984) Hyperadrenocorticism. *Vet. Clin. N. Am.* **14**, 731.

Richards M. A. (1974) The diabetes insipidus syndrome in dogs. In: Kirk R. W. (ed.), *Current Veterinary Therapy* V. Philadelphia, Saunders.

Roth J. A., Lomax L. G. Altszuler N. et al. (1980) Thymic abnormalities and growth hormone deficiency in dogs. *Am. J. Vet. Res.* **41**, 1256.

Scherding R. G., Meuten D. J., Chew D. J. et al. (1980) Primary hypoparathyroidism in the dog: a case report. *J. Am. Vet. Assoc.* **176**, 439.

Twedt D. C. and Wheeler S. L. (1984) Pheochromocytoma in the dog. *Vet. Clin. N. Am.* **14**, 767.

Weller R. E., Cullen J. and Dagle G. E. (1985) Hyperparathyroid disorders in the dog: primary, secondary and cancer-associated (pseudo). *J. Small Anim. Pract.* **26**, 329.

Chapter 37

Disorders of the
Female Genital Tract

(See also Jones and Joshua, 1982)

A. OVARIAN DISORDERS

1. Functional disturbances *(may also result from neoplasia)*
Pseudocyesis—'false pregnancy'
Very common in adult bitches, especially in middle age. Hormonal
problem, rather than psychological—luteal phase 1–3 months post-
oestrus—a *normal* feature of metoestrus.

Signs
    a. Behaviour:
        i. Nursing cushions/slippers/'toys'.
        ii. Hiding in corners, under beds.
        iii. Bed making.
    b. Temperament changes: aggression, restlessness *or*
        overaffection/clinging/lethargy.
    c. Anorexia (or polyphagia!).
    d. Mammary enlargement—may produce milk.
    e. May show full labour signs:
        trembling, whimpering, panting, licking genitalia.

Investigations check—
    a. That it is not a true pregnancy:
        i. Any chance of mating?
        ii. Abdominal palpation—negative?
        iii. Radiology (6–9 weeks) to check.
    b. That it is not pyometra (check with radiology?)
    N.B. There may be cystic endometrial hyperplasia.

225

Treatment

Is it necessary?—dogs will normally recover within a few weeks. If treated, suppression may only be temporary—the disorder may recur.

   a. Hormonal:
- i. Oestrogens (luteolytic):
  Stilboestrol 1–2 mg/day for 5 days.
  Oestradiol (Intervet) 0·5–1·0 mg s.c. for 5 days.
- ii. Progestogens (feed-back):
  Megestrol (Ovarid; Glaxo) 2 mg/kg for 5 days.
- iii. Androgens (antagonistic):
  Testosterone (1 mg/kg body weight for 5 days).
- iv. Mixture (e.g. Sesoral; Intervet).
- v. Prostaglandin F2α (50–100 µg/kg)—with CARE (toxic).

   But very likely to relapse.
   Avoid treatment if there is *any* chance of pregnancy.

   b. Sedatives, e.g. phenobarbitone, especially if anorexia or aggression is present.

   c. Diuresis or magnesium sulphate (Epsom salts).

   d. Ovariohysterectomy? if the problem is persistent or recurrent. Must be carried out when not lactating, or signs may persist.

Ovarian 'imbalance'

(poorly understood disorders) (Muller, Kirk and Scott, 1983)

Type I (mature entire bitches)—hyperoestrogenism.
→ Alopecia, (—and swelling of the perineum, vulva, nipples).
Often seborrhoea, anoestrus, irregular oestrus or false pregnancy.
Treatment. Ovariohysterectomy allows resolution—(often cystic ovaries).

Type II follows spaying when immature? (oestrogen-responsive).
→ Bilateral alopecia of the perineum, ears, ventral surfaces. Soft, thin skin and often a small vulva, incontinence.
Treatment. Usually responds to oestrogens (0·1–1·0 mg stilboestrol/ day, reducing).

Investigations
Difficult to confirm—test therapy is necessary.

Adult acromegaly
Progestogens induce growth hormone (*See* p. 204).

2. Ovarian tumours—often mixed:

    a. Granulosa cell/thecal (sex cord) tumour
    May → excess oestrogen
    Signs
        i. Prolonged oestrus, vulval swelling and haemorrhage, gynaecomastia, or other oestrus disturbances.
        ii. (Occasionally) anoestrus, false pregnancy or pyometra.
        iii. (Occasionally) large abdominal cystic mass.
    b. Cystadenoma (from coelomic epithelium)
    in mature, nulliparous bitches
    Signs
        i. Abdominal enlargement, pressure on other organs (rectum, bladder, etc.).
        ii. May seed, as carcinoma → abdominal neoplasia/ascites (Chapter 34).
    c. Dysgerminoma
    Found as a local swelling rather than malignancy (Chapter 34).

General treatment

Ovariohysterectomy and submit material for histopathology (for prognosis).

3. Ovarian cysts

    a. Cystadenoma—*see above* (B2).
    b. Luteal/follicular cysts—usually small and unimportant.

B. UTERINE DISORDERS

1. Pyometra

Due to defective reception or metabolism of normal hormones. Common in bitches over 6 years old: occasionally younger, and even in the uterine remnants of spayed bitches.

    A disease of metoestrus—may be a prolongation of oestrus.
                    —induced by cyclic oestrogen ↔ progestogen changes.

May be induced by:
    a. Use of oestrogens for misalliance at oestrus.
    b. Prolonged or excessive use of progestogens.

Signs

Not usually as serious if the cervix is *open* as if *closed:*
    a. Open pyometra: purulent vaginal discharge, may be an extension of pro-oestral bleeding.

  b. Closed pyometra:
    i. Signs of toxaemia: depression, pyrexia, anorexia, vomiting, polydipsia, polyuria, dehydration.
    ii. Abdominal enlargement?

Findings (not specific)
  a. Dehydration, elevation or depression of temperature.
  b. Abdominal pain?
  c. Palpably enlarged uterus?

Investigations
  a. Radiography is very useful in closed cases.
  b. Haematology—sometimes gross leucocytosis with a left shift.
        —occasionally anaemia, thrombocytopenia.
  c. Urinalysis—dilute; protein and casts may be present.
  d. Plasma urea may rise—often renal damage.

Treatment
Ovariohysterectomy following intravenous *fluid therapy.*
Prostaglandins *may* work, but *toxic* in dogs (Jones and Joshua, 1982).

2. Other genital tract disorders (*see* Jones and Joshua, 1982)

REFERENCES AND FURTHER READING

Greene J. A., Richardson R. C., Thornhill J. A. et al. (1979) Ovarian papillary cystadenocarcinoma in a bitch: case report and literature review. *J. Am. Anim. Hosp. Assoc.* **15**, 351.

Hardy R. M. and Osborne C. A. (1974) Canine pyometra: pathophysiology, diagnosis and treatment of uterine and extra-uterine lesions. *J. Am. Anim. Hosp. Assoc.* **10**, 245.

Jackson P. S., Furr B. J. A. and Hutchinson F. G. (1982) A preliminary study of pregnancy termination in the bitch with slow-release formulations of prostaglandin analogues *J. Small Anim. Pract.* **23**, 287.

Jones D. E. and Joshua J. O. (1982) *Reproductive Clinical Problems in the Dog.* Bristol, Wright PSG.

Muller G. H., Kirk R. W. and Scott D. W. (1983) *Small Animal Dermatology.* Philadelphia, Saunders.

Olson P. N., Husted P. W., Allen T. A. and Nett T. M. (1984) Reproductive endocrinology and physiology of the bitch and queen. *Vet. Clin. N. Am.* **14**, 927.

Sokolowski J. H. (1980) Prostaglandin F_2 Alpha-THAM for medical treatment of endometritis, metritis and pyometritis in the bitch. *J. Am. Anim. Hosp. Assoc.* **16**, 119.

Chapter 38

Differential Diagnosis of Polydipsia

Thirst is influenced by many factors, particularly endocrine balance, and transient increases in thirst are common in dogs for no immediately obvious reason. Increasing awareness of the potential significance of polydipsia among clients means that many cases now presented with a history of recent polydipsia may have no significant disease revealed by investigation.

Normal dogs:
1. Usually drink less than 100 ml/kg body weight/day.
2. Produce less urine than 50 ml/kg body weight/day.

CAUSES OF POLYDIPSIA

1. Polyuria

Due to:
- *a.* Endocrine disturbances:
  - i. Diabetes mellitus.
  - ii. Diabetes insipidus.
  - iii. Hyperadrenocorticalism.
  - iv. (Hyperthyroidism.)
  - v. (Hyperparathyroidism.)
  - vi. Adult acromegaly.
  - vii. (Hypoadrenocorticalism)
- *b.* Renal dysfunction:
  - i. Renal failure (compensated/decompensating).
  - ii. Toxaemic immune damage:
    Pyometra.
    Hepatic
    Sepsis.

             iii. Adaptation to chronic polydipsia (e.g. psychogenic).
      c. Hepatic failure
      d. Iatrogenic causes:
             i. Glucocorticoids.
             ii. Diuretics (frusemide/thiazides/xanthines).
             iii. Progestogens, thyroid and other hormones.
      e. Primary renal glycosuria (including Fanconi syndrome).

2. Other excess fluid loss

      a. Diarrhoea/vomiting.
      b. Pyogenic foci (pyometra, pyothorax).
      c. Effusions (thorax/abdomen).
      d. Haemorrhage.
      e. Lactation.

3. Environmental

      a. Diet—dry or semi-moist foods, high salt content.
      b. Central heating, hot weather.
      c. Heavy exercise.

4. Psychogenic

5. Other (including hepatic failure and congestive cardiac failure).

INVESTIGATION OF POLYDIPSIA

1. *History:*
      a. Speed of onset.
      b. Changes in environment and diet.
      c. Oestrus history.
      d. Urinary function.
      e. Other signs of disease (*see* 2).
2. *Clinical signs:*
      a. Hyperadrenocorticalism:
         dropped abdomen, alopecia, weakness and polyphagia.
      b. Diabetes mellitus:
         polyphagia, weight loss, mainly in middle-aged bitches.
      c. Pyometra: toxaemia, vaginal discharge.
      d. Diabetes insipidus:
         enormous thirst, dehydration?; the dog is otherwise *well*.
      e. Renal failure: weight loss, depression, partial anorexia.

3. *Quantitate:*
Persuade the client to measure the water intake, or admit the dog to kennels to measure water over a few days.
4. If thirst is genuinely excessive—
Collect urine for analysis:
   a. If well concentrated (> 1·025 s.g.) check for glucose = diabetes mellitus or other disorders (p. 217)?
   b. If s.g. < 1·025:
      i. Check plasma urea—chronic renal failure?
      ii. Check plasma glucose, haematology = diabetes mellitus, hyperadrenocorticalism?
      iii. Re-check urinalysis.
      iv. Check liver enzymes: if raised = hyperadrenocorticalism/hepatopathy?
5. If no clear-cut diagnosis—
Conduct a *Water Deprivation Test:*
   a. Starve the dog for 12 hours,
      —remove and withhold water overnight.
   b. Empty the bladder (catheter?) and weigh dog in the morning.
   c. Re-catheterize 2–4 hourly and re-weigh
      Check urine s.g.
   d. Stop $\left\{\begin{array}{l}\text{if the dog is dehydrated.}\\ \text{when weight loss reaches 5 per cent.}\\ \text{if urine s.g. concentrates} > 1\cdot025.\\ (= \text{normal dog/psychogenic polydipsia?}).\end{array}\right.$

N.B. *Never* conduct this test if the plasma urea is elevated.
Typical urine concentrations (variable):
   a. 1·020–1·040 normal dog (but a normal dog can produce urine of between 1·001–1·065 according to state of hydration).
   b. 1·002–1·008 diabetes insipidus (or psychogenic polydipsia).
   c. 1·004–1·010 hyperadrenocorticalism (but will concentrate if dehydrated).
   d. 1·008–1·018 chronic renal failure.
   e. > 1·030 diabetes mellitus.
6. If urine unconcentrated, may be:
   a. Non-uraemic renal compensation.
   b. Diabetes insipidus (true or nephrogenic).
   c. Renal adaptation to psychogenic polydipsia.
   d. Hyperadrenocorticalism?
Then try *ADH response test:*
(N.B. Pitressin tannate in oil is now unavailable.)
      i. Empty the bladder and prepare as for water deprivation test (as in 5).
      ii. Inject desmopressin (DDAVP; Ferring) 0·3–1·0 ml i.m.

   iii. Collect urine after 6 hours, re-weigh and check as in (5).

   'Cranial' diabetes insipidus ⎱ should concentrate.
   Hyperadrenocorticalism ⎰

   N.B. *Never* conduct this test if the plasma urea is elevated.

7. If still no concentration:
   Renal adaptation or nephrogenic diabetes insipidus àre possible diagnoses.
   Perform *Hickey Hare Test?*
     a. Give 20 ml/kg body weight of water by stomach tube.
     b. Administer 2·5 per cent NaCl (10 mg/kg) i.v. by slow drip.
     c. Monitor urine production:
       i. Decreases in renal adaptation.
       ii. Unaltered in nephrogenic diabetes insipidus.

N.B. Plasma and urine osmolalities are the *best* way to assess concentration (osmolality is measured by the depression in freezing point of the fluid)—they represent the number of particles of solute (Osborne, Low and Finco, 1972). However, osmolality is not easily assessed in practice.

Normal plasma: 300 mosm/kg
Normal urine: 500–1500 mosm/kg (> 2000 with dehydration)
Diabetes insipidus ⎱   < 250 mosm/kg urine (< *plasma*)
Renal adaptation   ⎰   (also in overhydration or diuresis)

Urine elevates ⎸× 2–10 with ADH response test (nephrogenic diabetes insipidus → no change).

FURTHER READING

Hardy R. M. and Osborne C. A. (1978) Water deprivation test in the dog: maximal normal values. *J. Am. Vet. Med. Assoc.* **174**, 479.

Hardy R. M. and Osborne C. A. (1980) Water deprivation and vasopressin concentration tests in the differentiation of polyuric syndromes. In: Kirk R. W. (ed.) *Current Veterinary Therapy VII.* Philadelphia, Saunders.

Mackenzie C. P. and van den Broek A. (1982) The Fanconi syndrome in a whippet. *J. Small Anim. Pract.* **23**, 469.

Mulnix J. A., Rijnberk A. and Hendriks H. J. (1976) Evaluation of a modified water-deprivation test for diagnosis of polyuric disorders in dogs. *J. Am. Vet. Med. Assoc.* **169**, 1327.

Osborne C. A. (1970) Urologic logic—diagnosis of renal disease. *J. Am. Vet. Med. Assoc.* **157**, 1656.

Osborne C. A., Low D. G. and Finco D. R. (1972) *Canine and Feline Urology.* Philadelphia, Saunders.

Richards M. A. (1969) The differential diagnosis of polyuric syndromes in the dog. *J. Small Anim. Pract.* **10**, 651.

Chapter 39

Differential Diagnosis of Thinness and Weight Loss

1. Diet:
    a. Insufficient quantity.
    b. Poor quality, especially working Collies fed only grain.
    c. Vitamin D toxicity.
2. Dysphagia or inappetance (dental disorders, oropharyngeal lesions).
3. Persistent vomiting or regurgitation of food (Chapter 19).
4. Maldigestion or malabsorption (Chapter 21).
5. Toxaemias:
    a. Renal failure (Chapter 28).
    b. Hepatic failure (Chapter 24).
    c. Septic focus (pyometra, pyothorax, prostatic abscess).
    d. Iatrogenic (e.g. cardiac glycosides).
6. Neoplasia:
    a. Carcinomata:
        i. Generalized.
        ii. Mammary.
        iii. Pulmonary.
        iv. Gastrointestinal.
        v. Abdominal (hepatic/pancreatic).
    b. Lymphosarcoma.
    c. Leukaemia.
    d. Other generalized disseminated tumours.
7. Metabolic/endocrine disorders (Chapter 36):
    a. Diabetes mellitus.
    b. Hypoadrenocorticalism.
    c. Hyperthyroidism (rare).
    d. Hyperparathyroidism.

8. Sepsis (urinary, thoracic, abdominal, endocarditis).
9. Idiopathic/psychological disorders:
    a. Certain breeds may be naturally very thin
       (German Shepherd/Irish Setter/Afghan).
    b. Nervous dogs (often similar breeds).
10. Parasitism (external or alimentary).
11. High levels of exercise, pregnancy, lactation
    (may each require massive increases in dietary intake).
12. Protein loss (enteropathy, glomerulonephritis).

INVESTIGATION OF THINNESS AND WEIGHT LOSS

History

    a. Diet/appetite/exercise.
    b. Weight *loss*—or natural physique?
    c. Vomiting/regurgitation? (obstruction?)
    d. Diarrhoea/bulky faeces? (malabsorption?)
    e. Polydipsia? (endocrine or renal disease?)
    f. Other signs—cough or dyspnoea?

Findings

    a. Body weight—*weigh* the dog and *record.*
    b. Thin body but well muscled?
    c. Neoplasia? (especially check lymph nodes, abdomen).
    d. Signs of toxaemia? (renal).
    e. Signs of pallor or jaundice.
    f. Evidence of serous cavity effusions?
    g. Pyrexia? (Chapter 41).

Investigations

    a. Check the diet—change if incorrect.
    b. Weigh the dog.
    c. Feed the corrected diet for 1–2 weeks.
    d. Re-weigh the dog.
    If no weight gain:
    e. Check whether there is any vomiting or diarrhoea.
    f. Check the water intake (Chapter 38).
    g. Check:
        i. Plasma/urea/glucose/liver enzymes.
        ii. Routine haematology.

   iii. Biochemistry:
        Proteins.
        Calcium/phosphorus (parathyroid?).
        Sodium/potassium (adrenal?).
   iv. Urinalysis.
   h. Radiograph the thorax for neoplasms?
If no abnormality:
   i. Feed an increased diet for 1–2 weeks.
   j. Re-weigh the dog after increasing the food intake.
   k. Admit the dog to kennels, re-assess and observe.
   l. Investigate any body system implicated by signs.
   m. Use tests for malabsorption (Chapter 21).

DIFFERENTIAL DIAGNOSIS FOR OBESITY

Hypothyroidism (*see* p. 206)—but many cases are not obese.
Hyperadrenocorticalism (*see* p. 212)—large abdomen.
Adult acromegaly or latent diabetes mellitus (Chapter 36).
Other causes of abdominal enlargement (Chapter 34).
Pituitary or hypothalamic disorders.

Check

   a. Thyroid hormone levels.
   b. Plasma cortisol.
   c. Glucose tolerance test.

Treatment

Intake of fats should be reduced as much as possible—especially in meat trimmings and scraps from plates. Some biscuit or meal should be withdrawn in favour of *fibre.*
N.B.: Dogs can survive starvation for weeks without developing ketoacidosis or severe hypoproteinaemia.

FURTHER READING

Andersen G. L. and Lewis L. D. (1980) Obesity. In: Kirk R. W. (ed.) *Current Veterinary Therapy* VII Philadelphia, Saunders.

Chapter 40

Autoimmune Disorders

Numerous disorders have now been discovered—'collagen diseases'—in which circulating antibodies are directed against the host's own tissues. Aetiology and details of many disorders are not fully understood. These disorders *may* be initiated by various drugs, toxins, neoplasia or infections. They may occur in combination, e.g. as systemic lupus erythematosus (SLE). Often found in young adult bitches.

A. AUTOIMMUNE HAEMOLYTIC ANAEMIA

a. Intravascular—acute agglutination or haemolysis.
b. Extravascular → decreased RBC lifespan—a slower process. RBC are withdrawn in the spleen, liver, bone marrow.

Signs (usually sudden onset)

a. Depression, anorexia (dyspnoea).
b. Weakness, lethargy. Can be temperature-dependent, e.g. in cold weather.

Findings

a. Pale mucous membranes, weak pulse.
b. Tachycardia.
c. Sometimes: lymphadenopathy, splenomegaly, hepatomegaly.
d. Occasionally: icterus, haemoglobinuria if intravascular.

Investigations

  a. Routine haematology:
     i. Regenerative anaemia.
     ii. Spherocytosis, schistocytosis.
     iii. Reticulocytosis, anisocytosis.
     iv. May be autoagglutination.
  b. Coombs' test positive—*but* false positives can occur.
                    —use freshly washed cells.
  c. Papain test positive (Jones and Darke, 1975).

Treatment

  a. High levels of corticosteroids (2–5 mg/kg prednisolone daily)
     Beware
     i. Uraemia—if also glomerulonephritis/renal insufficiency.
     ii. Secondary infections.
     iii. Hepatic involvement (steroid hepatopathy).
  b. Splenectomy?—may reduce the rate of RBC withdrawal,
     especially if no response to *a*.
  c. Transfusion?
     But—may *accelerate* haemolysis.
        —transfused RBC are very rapidly removed from the
        circulation in most cases.
     Therefore:
     i. Use only if critical (PCV <10 per cent).
     ii. Important to cross-match bloods (Chapter 42).
  d. Salicylates, phenylbutazone
     (anti-inflammatory and anti-pyretics).
  e. Other immunosuppressants?: azathioprine (2 mg/kg daily);
     cyclophosphamide (2 mg/kg daily for 4 days per week).
     And *check* haematology for marrow depression.

B. AUTOIMMUNE THROMBOCYTOPENIA

Signs

Purpura—bruising, haemorrhages, weakness, lethargy.
May be associated with other autoimmune disorders.

Findings

Bruising, pale mucous membranes, ecchymoses (lymphadenopathy,
splenomegaly), other sites of blood loss?

Investigations

   a. Haematology—regenerative anaemia (Chapter 42).
              —profound thrombocytopenia ($<50\,000/mm^3$).
   b. Prolonged bleeding time.
   c. Poor clot retraction in a clotted sample.
   d. Platelet Factor 3 released (if it can be assessed).

Other causes of persistent bleeding (Chapter 42)

   a. Iatrogenic thrombocytopenia.
   b. Thrombasthenia.
   c. Idiopathic thrombocytopenia.
   d. Thrombocythaemia.
   e. Coagulopathies.
   f. Vasculitis.
   g. Neoplasia.

Treatment

As for autoimmune haemolytic anaemia.

C. SYSTEMIC LUPUS ERYTHEMATOSUS (SLE)

Associated with anti-DNA antibody. Immune complexes → tissues.
Combination of one or more multi-systemic disorders;
1. Polyarthritis.
2. Haemolytic anaemia.
3. Thrombocytopenia.
4. Glomerulonephritis.
5. Skin lesions—erythema, eczematous reaction.
6. Occasionally: polymyositis, pleurisy, lymphomegaly.

Signs

Very variable:
   a. Stiffness, anorexia, lethargy.
   b. Occasionally: CNS disturbances.

Findings

   a. Pyrexia, pallor.
   b. Lymphadenopathy, splenomegaly.
   c. Joint pain.

Investigations

Specialist tests (Bennett, 1980):
  a. LE cell preparation is usually positive.
  b. Antinuclear antibody test is usually positive.
  c. Gammaglobulin levels are high.
  d. Haemolytic anaemia, thrombocytopenia, leucopenia?
  e. Positive Coombs' test?
  f. Biopsy—kidneys, joint synovia: complement may be identified in some tissues.

Treatment

Corticosteroids, salicylates, immunosuppression? (*see* p. 237).

D. OTHER DISORDERS

1. Autoimmune polyarthritis.
2. Polyarteritis/periarteritis nodosa.
3. Glomerulonephritis.
4. Rheumatoid arthritis.

E. OTHER DISEASES WITH PROVEN IMMUNE-MEDIATED COMPONENTS

1. Lymphocytic thyroiditis.
2. Myasthenia gravis.
3. Pemphigus vulgaris, bullous pemphigoid.
4. Distemper demyelination.
5. Chronic active hepatitis.

REFERENCES AND FURTHER READING

Bennett D. (1980) Autoimmune disease in the dog. In: Yoxall A. T. and Hird J. P. R. (ed.), *Physiological Basis of Small Animal Practice.* Oxford, Blackwell Scientific.

Bennett D., Finnett S. L., Nash A. S. et al. (1981) Primary autoimmune haemolytic anaemia in the dog. *Vet. Rec.* **109**, 150.

Dodds W. J. (1977) Autoimmune hemolytic disease and other causes of immune-mediated anemia: an overview. *J. Am. Anim. Hosp. Assoc.* **13**, 437.

Grindem C. B. and Johnson K. H. (1983) Systemic lupus erythematosus: literature review and report of 42 new cases. *J. Am. Anim. Hosp. Assoc.* **19**, 489.

Jones D. R. E. and Darke P. G. G. (1975) Use of papain for the detection of incomplete erythrocyte auto-antibodies in autoimmune haemolytic anaemia of the dog and cat. *J. Small Anim. Pract.* **16**, 273.

Newton C. D., Lipowitz A. F., Halliwell R. E. W. et al. (1976) Rheumatoid arthritis in dogs. *J. Am. Vet. Med. Assoc.* **168**, 113.

Randell M. G. and Hurvitz A. I. (1983) Immune-mediated vasculitis in five dogs. *J. Am. Vet. Med. Assoc.* **183**, 207.

Werner L. L. and Halliwell R. E. W. (1984) Diseases associated with autoimmunity. In: Chandler E. A., Sutton J. B. and Thompson D. J. (eds.) *Canine Medicine and Therapeutics,* 2nd Ed. Oxford, Blackwell.
Wilkins R. J., Hurvitz A. I. and Dodds-Laffin W. J. (1973) Immunologically mediated thrombocytopenia in the dog. *J. Am. Vet. Med. Assoc.* **163**, 277.
Williams D. A. and Maggio-Price L. (1984) Canine idiopathic thrombocytopenia: clinical observations and long-term follow up in 54 cases. *J. Am. Vet. Med. Assoc.* **185**, 660.

Chapter 41

Differential Diagnosis of Recurrent or Persistent Pyrexia

Pyrexia of unknown origin (PUO) is a relatively common problem in small animal practice, presenting a diagnostic challenge. Many causes of persistent pyrexia and leucocytosis are *not* associated with bacterial infection. If antibiotics are indicated, they may be required for weeks. They are *not* antipyretic agents.

AETIOLOGY

1. Infections

   a. Bite wounds, cellulitis, dental sepsis.
   b. Foreign body abscesses:
      i. Superficial.
      ii. Deep—oesphageal, pharyngeal, or intestinal penetrations.
         —body cavities (→ serous cavity effusions).
   c. Endocarditis (and myocarditis).
   d. Internal sepsis: pyometra, bronchopneumonia, pericarditis, pleurisy, peritonitis (especially nocardiosis).
   e. Urinary infections: pyelonephritis, prostatitis.
   f. Osteomyelitis.
   g. Persistent viral infections (immunosuppression?).
   h. Other infections: toxoplasmosis, brucellosis, tuberculosis, mycosis.
   i. Post-surgical infection.
   j. Cyclic neutropenia (Collies), other WBC disturbances.

2. Inflammation/tissue necrosis

   a. Subperiosteal haemorrhage (hypertrophic osteodystrophy).
   b. Encephalitis, intracranial tumours or trauma.

  c. Neoplastic reaction or necrosis—especially with:
    i. Lymphosarcoma.
    ii. Leukaemias.
    iii. Myeloma.
    iv. Carcinomata.
    v. Hepatic neoplasia.
  d. Infarcted tissues, organ torsion (testis, spleen).

3. Autoimmune and collagenous disorders (Chapter 40)

  a. Systemic lupus erythematosus.
  b. Rheumatoid arthritis.
  c. Polyarteritis/periarteritis nodosa.
  d. (Autoimmune haemolytic anaemia or thrombocytopenia).

4. Metabolic/endocrine disorders (Chapter 36)

Hyperthyroidism, phaeochromocytoma.

5. Other disorders

Idiopathic, pain, fear.

INVESTIGATION OF PERSISTENT OR RECURRENT PYREXIA

History

Previous wounds, injuries, surgery?
Signs of system involvement—alimentary, respiratory, urinary?

Signs

  a. *Depression,* anorexia and lethargy are usual.
  b. Stiffness, lameness and dyspnoea are also common.
  c. Specific organ or system involvement (sepsis/neoplasia)?
N.B. Active and excitable dogs readily produce a 'surgery' pyrexia.

Findings

  a. Rectal temperature remains persistently above 39·0°C.
  b. Joint or other pain? (polyarthritis, polyarteritis).
  c. Cardiac murmur? rapid change in character? (endocarditis)
    dysrhythmia? (myocarditis).

But a murmur may be secondary to anaemia or
   hypoproteinaemia.
 d. Pleural or abdominal effusions?
 e. Enlargement of any organ?
 f. Examine and *re-examine* for changes.

Investigations

 a. Record the temperature and pulse twice daily.
 b. Routine haematology:
     i. Leucocytosis? left shift?
     ii. Leukaemia?
     iii Anaemia?
     and *repeat* sample frequently.
But leucocytosis occurs in many cases of PUO, however caused.
 c. Plasma proteins—gammaglobulins are raised in sepsis/
    inflammatory/necrotic/autoimmune disorders.
 d. Blood culture:
     i. May need to be repeated several times for success.
     ii. Must have received *no* antibiotics for 7 days.
     iii Best taken at the time of maximal pyrexia.
 e. Radiology:
     i. Evidence of pleural or abdominal effusions or abscesses?
     ii. Evidence of *neoplasia?*
     iii. Evidence of bone necrosis?
 f. Urine:
     i. Pus or haematuria (microscopic?).
     ii. Cells (neoplastic?).
 g. ECG for dysrhythmias (Chapter 11).
 h. Autoimmune tests (Chapter 40).
 i. *Biopsy* may be indicated:
     i. Bone marrow, lymph nodes, any enlarged organ.
     ii. Aspirate fluids (serous cavities, joints).

Treatment

Only when a diagnosis has been achieved:
 a. Sepsis:
     High levels of antibiotics.
     —Several times daily.
     —For several weeks.
 b. Autoimmune disorders:
     i. Corticosteroids at high doses (Chapter 40).

    c. Antipyretics:
       i. Salicylates (aspirin 30 mg/kg t.d.s.).
      ii. Phenothiazine derivatives (acepromazine).
N.B. Symptomatic treatment often masks further symptoms, and may be counterproductive, in precluding a definitive diagnosis.

FURTHER READING

Chiapella A. M. (1980) Fevers of unknown origin in dogs and cats. In: Kirk R. W. (ed.), *Current Veterinary Therapy VII.* Philadelphia, Saunders.
Davis L E. (1979) Fever. *J. Am. Vet. Med. Assoc.* **175**, 1210.
Michell A. R. (1982) Current concepts of fever. *J. Small Anim. Pract.* **23**, 185.

Chapter 42

Anaemia

(More correctly: oligaemia)

A clinical sign, not a specific diagnosis. Treatment must therefore be directed towards the specific cause; iron and vitamin B_{12}, though commonly used, are very rarely required.

A. ACUTE HAEMORRHAGE (internal or external)

1. Trauma or surgery.
2. Coagulation disorders:
    a. Warfarin poisoning.
    b. Hepatic failure (Chapter 24).
    c. Disseminated intravascular coagulation (DIC) or thrombosis (paradoxically → haemorrhage). (Greene, 1975.)
    d. Haemophilias (young dogs) (Factors VII–X).
3. Bleeding disorders:
    a. Thrombocytopenia:
        i. Autoimmune.
        ii. Idiopathic.
        iii. Iatrogenic marrow depression (salicylates, phenylbutazone, oestrogens, phenothiazines, sulphonamides, phenytoin).
        iv. Marrow depression in infection/neoplasia.
        v. Splenic sequestration of platelets.
    b. Platelet malfunction or neoplasia (thrombasthenia, thrombocythaemia).
4. Neoplastic erosion of blood vessels:
    Haemangiosarcoma (spleen, liver, lungs).
    Can cause repeated haemorrhage into body cavities or lungs (Chapters 3 and 34).

5. Vasculitis:
   a. Canine viral hepatitis.
   b. Immune polyarteritis.
   c. *Angiostrongylus vasorum.*
6. Other disorders causing intestinal haemorrhage (Chapter 22).

Signs

   a. Collapse/weakness/lethargy.
   b. Dyspnoea.

Findings (*see* p. 250)

   a. Pallor, tachycardia.
   b. Initially a normal blood picture, later: regenerative anaemia.
   c. Recurrent or persistent haemorrhage may cause hypoplastic anaemia and reduced plasma proteins.
   d. Prolonged clotting/bleeding/prothrombin time? (p. 254).
   e. Fibrin degradation products elevated?

Specific treatment (*see also* p. 251)

   a. Plasma expander/intravenous fluids/blood transfusion? (*see* p. 252).
   b. Vitamin K₁ (Konakion; Roche)—if Warfarin (1 mg/kg body weight for 5 days).
   c. Corticosteroids (hypovolaemic shock, thrombocytopenia or immune disease)?
   d. Exploratory laparotomy? If a possibility of neoplasia (following fluid replacement).

B. CHRONIC BLOOD LOSS

1. Haematuria (Chapter 31):
   a. Cystitis.
   b. Calculi.
   c. Tumours (bladder, urethra, kidney).
   d. Prostatic disorders (Chapter 30).
   e. Uterine disorders.
2. Epistaxis:
   a. Nasal neoplasia.
   b. Rhinitis (Aspergillus/other).
3. Melaena:
   a. Peptic ulcer/neoplasm.
   b. Intussusception (partial obstruction).

4. Fresh blood in faeces (*see* Chapter 22):
    a. Colitis/proctitis.
    b. Neoplasia.
    c. Foreign body.
    d. Intussusception (colonic).
5. Parasitic infection:
    a. Ectoparasites—fleas, lice (if severe).
    b. Hookworms (uncommonly in UK).
6. Bleeding disorders (as A3)

Findings

Microcytic, hypochromic anaemia (hypoplastic) (p. 250).
Reduced serum iron concentration?

Specific treatment

a. Eliminate the source of haemorrhage.
b. Attend to nutritional intake and consider transfusion (p. 251).

C. TOXAEMIC/INVASIVE MARROW DEPRESSION

(May also cause increased RBC fragility and shortened lifespan)

1. Toxaemia: chronic renal or hepatic failure.
2. Chronic suppuration (Endocarditis, pyothorax, pyometra.)
3. Malignant haemopoietic neoplasia
   (Leukaemia, myeloma, lymphosarcoma, metastases.)
4. Endocrine disorders (Hypothyroidism, hypoadrenocorticalism, hyperoestrogenism.)
5. Iatrogenic
   (Oestrogens, chloramphenicol, phenytoin, phenylbutazone.)
6. Poisoning (lead, arsenic).
7. Immune-mediated
8. Idiopathic.

Usually other major signs of disease occur simultaneously.

Findings

a. Little regeneration (p. 250). Low reticulocyte count.
b. Normocytic, normochromic anaemia
   (microcytic, hypochromic ± basophilic stippling in lead poisoning).
c. Other marrow-produced cells may be low (platelets, WBC).

Determine the cause.

Treatment (supportive)

   a. *Treat the cause*—every effort should be made.
   b. Anabolic steroids.
   c. Good nutrition (complete, meat diet).
   d. Blood transfusion? (*see* p. 252).
   e. Corticosteroids? (as immunosuppressants).

D. HAEMOLYSIS

1. Autoimmune haemolytic anaemia (Chapter 40).
2. Other haemolytic anaemias:
   a. Isoimmune (in pups from transfused dams).
   b. Pyruvate kinase deficiency (Basenjis).
   c. Leptospirosis or streptococcal infection?
   d. Idiopathic—a number of cases are unaccountable.
   e. Babesia, haemobartonella, leishmaniasis (imported).
   f. Increased RBC fragility in toxaemias/heat stroke/radiation.

Findings

   a. Jaundice or haemoglobinuria is unusual in dogs.
   b. Regeneration + + + : normoblasts, reticulocytes.
   c. Macrocytic, hypochromic anaemia.
   d. Spherocytes, schistocytes may be present (autoimmune disease).
   e. Often also evidence of WBC regeneration.

Specific treatment

   a. Corticosteroids at high dose rates (prednisolone 2–5 mg/kg/day)?—for autoimmune haemolysis.
   b. Splenectomy?
   c. Antibiotics for infections.

E. NUTRITIONAL MARROW DEFICIENCY (uncommon)

1. Iron deficiency: usually *secondary* to:
   a. Chronic haemorrhage.
   b. Malabsorption, maldigestion.
   c. Generalized disease in young pups.
2. B vitamin deficiency (B_6, B_{12}, folic acid)
   a. Malabsorption, maldigestion.
   b. Hepatic failure? Phenytoin toxicity.
3. Marrow exhaustion (in chronic regeneration).

Findings

Non-regenerative anaemia (p. 250):
  a. Microcytic, hypochromic, but normal reticulocytes.
  b. (Macrocytic in vitamin B_{12} deficiency—*rare*).
  c. Low serum iron level (< 60 mg %)?

Specific treatment

According to anticipated cause:
Iron: ferrous sulphate 5 mg/kg body weight i.m.

INVESTIGATION OF ANAEMIA

Always try to establish a *cause*.
Symptomatic treatment is rarely of great value.

Types of anaemia

Haemorrhagic

Caused by:
  a. Vascular damage (trauma/neoplasia/vasculitis).
  b. Clotting defects (p. 245).
  c. Platelet dysfunction or thrombocytopenia.

Characteristics
  a. Normal haematology—for the first few hours.
  b. Regenerative pattern (2 days → weeks).
  c. Hypoplastic pattern (if chronic or recurrent).
  d. Abnormal coagulation test results? (p. 254).
  e. A fall in plasma proteins and platelets in acute haemorrhage.

Haemolytic

Caused by:
  a. Autoimmune disease.
  b. Toxins, radiation, heat stroke?
  c. (Parasitic infections.)

Characteristics
  a. Regenerative pattern and spherocytes, schistocytes?
  b. (Prehepatic jaundice, haemoglobinuria—uncommon in dogs.)
  c. Leucocytosis.

Hypoplastic

Caused by:
  a. Toxic marrow depression (toxaemic, endocrine, iatrogenic).

    b. Marrow invasion (neoplastic or leukaemic).
    c. Nutritional deficiency (*uncommon* in dogs).

Characteristics
    a. Hypoplastic pattern.
    b. Also thrombocytopenia, granulocytopenia?

Erythrocyte patterns in anaemia
    a. Regeneration:
       i. Presence of immature RBCs (after a few days):
          reticulocytes, normoblasts (when severe)
      ii. Evidence of immaturity of RBCs:
          anisocytosis, polychromasia, macrocytic pattern.
      iii. Evidence of other hyperplasia—thrombocytosis,
           leucocytosis?
      iv. High mean corpuscular volume (MCV).
    b. Hypoplasia:
       i. Normal pattern (normocytic, normochromic)
         —with low RBC count, no reticulocytes.
      ii. Microcytic, hypochromic (low MCV, MCHC)
         —(if iron depletion in chronic disease).
      iii. Evidence of other marrow depression?
         —granulocytopenia, thrombocytopenia.

History

    a. Duration and acuteness.
    b. Possibility of trauma/drugs/toxins?
    c. Any signs of recent haemorrhage? (Check all sites).

General signs

    a. Lethargy, weakness, collapse.
    b. Dyspnoea (or syncope) with exertion.

Findings

    a. Pallor, weak pulse (tapping or variable).
       N.B. Pallor does *not* always represent anaemia
       —it is affected also by the circulation.
    b. Tachycardia ± systolic murmur (haemic).
    c. Examine all sites for haemorrhage
       Mucous membranes, rectum, mouth, abdomen, thorax,
       joints, skin, urine.
    d. Splenomegaly, lymphomegaly, hepatomegaly.
       (Neoplasia, leukaemia, autoimmune disorder?)

Further investigations

a. Check routine haematology,
and *monitor* closely day by day:
  i. Determine whether *regenerative* or *hypoplastic* pattern.
  ii. How severely anaemic.
  ii. Platelet counts.
Prepare and dry a fresh blood smear
—as well as taking an EDTA sample.
b. If a haemorrhagic disorder, determine (p. 254):
  i. Clotting time (normally 4–10 min in plain tube).
  ii. Clot retraction—delayed in platelet disorders.
  iii. Bleeding time (normal < 5 min)—delayed in platelet disorders.
  iv. Other laboratory tests: prothrombin time (p. 255) liver enzymes (p. 149).
c. If a suggestion of autoimmune disease (Chapter 40)—try:
  i. Coombs' test.
  ii. Papain test.
  iii. Antinuclear antibody test.
But all require specialist laboratory assistance.
d. If a hypoplastic anaemia:
Try a marrow biopsy (specialist examination)
(Penny and Carlisle, 1970):
  i. Local analgesia and sterile preparation.
  ii. Incise skin dorsal to the iliac crest.
  iii. Introduce the biopsy needle into the ilium from above.
  iv. Use suction with a 20–ml syringe.
  v. Prepare immediate smears and stain (specialist).
e. If in any doubt about possible haemorrhage:
  i. Check urine for microscopic haematuria.
  ii. Check faeces for blood
—when no meat has been fed for 48 hours.
  iii. Check the body cavities, for haemorrhage.

Treatment

a. In acute anaemia (haemorrhagic, haemolytic) give:
  i. Corticosteroids (prednisolone: 2–5 mg/kg body weight).
  ii. Vitamin K_1 (Konakion; Roche)
1 mg/kg body weight/day for 5 days (i.v. or i.m.).
But very important to try to establish a *diagnosis* first.
b. To assist regeneration in chronic haemorrhage or hypoplasia:
  i. *Rest* and feed a good quality, high protein diet.
  ii. Administer B vitamins, anabolic steroids, folic acid.

    iii. ?Administer iron dextran 25 mg/kg body weight i.m.
  c. Consider *fluid therapy* in acute haemorrhage:
    especially plasma expanders (Haemaccel; Hoechst),
    rather than blood, if not immediately available.

Transfusions

Have a dramatic effect on the dog (and client!).
Uses:
  a. Weak, incapacitated animal (especially in chronic anaemia).
  b. Preparatory to surgery.
  c. Following traumatic or surgical haemorrhage.
  d. Following the loss of clotting factors or platelets.
    —especially if the PCV falls below 20 per cent.
But:
  a. They obscure the diagnosis.
  b. The dog may deteriorate again, despite transfusion.
  c. There is a likelihood of reaction if repetition is necessary.
  d. Transfused RBCs may be rapidly removed from the circulation
    of the recipient?
    (especially in autoimmune haemolytic anaemia.)

60 per cent of dogs are A-positive (universal recipients).
40 per cent of dogs are A-negative (universal donors).
Only presents a problem with repeat transfusions (in 15–25%?)
But cross-matching should be attempted if possible
(Crispin, 1981; O'Rourke, 1983).

Technique for transfusion
  a. Ensure sterility.
  b. Receive blood from the donor's jugular vein into CPD (citrate
    phosphate dextrose) (Travenol).
  c. Mix thoroughly with anticoagulant during collection.
  d. Store at 4–6 °C for a maximum of 4 weeks (for RBC).
    (Platelets and most clotting factors last < *2 days.*)
  e. Administer through a giving set with a filter
    —as fresh as possible
  f. Give 10–20 ml/kg, slowly, for chronic anaemia.
    Give according to rate of blood loss in acute haemorrhage.
Always consider fluid therapy as an alternative.

APPROACH TO UNACCOUNTABLE HAEMORRHAGE OR PROLONGED BLEEDING

Unexpected or prolonged bleeding may result from poor surgical
ligation, or from lesions such as neoplasms (p. 245). Warfarin poisoning,

while common, is often over-diagnosed as a cause of haemorrhage. Repeated bleeding should be investigated thoroughly.

History

    a. Any previous prolonged bleeding?
        Any problems followed previous trauma or surgery?
    b. Access to poisons?
        Possibility of trauma?
        Recent administration of drugs?
    c. Any related animals affected?
        Age at which signs were first seen? (congenital?)
    d. Large volume haemorrhage or purpural bruising?
        (clotting, platelet or vascular defect?)
    e. Site of haemorrhage: single or multiple?
        (Solitary *lesion* or coagulopathy?).
    f. Other sites affected?
        Check gums, nose, urine, faeces, joints, body cavities (petechiae, epistaxis, haematuria, melaena?).
    g. Immunization—leptospirosis or viral hepatitis?

Findings

    a. Pallor if severe anaemia.
    b. Petechiae, purpura, gum haemorrhage? (platelet or vascular disorder).
    c. Other evidence of haemorrhage: body cavities, joints? (coagulopathy).
    d. Other underlying disease?
    e. Check for:
        i. Hepatic failure, uraemia.
        ii. Autoimmune or immune-mediated disorders.
        iii. Malignancy, systemic infections.

Investigations

    a. Routine haematology:
        i. Regenerative anaemia initially.
        ii. Hypoplastic pattern if prolonged or recurrent haemorrhage.
    b. Try to assess whether the haemorrhage is due to:
        i. True clotting defect.
        ii. Platelet dysfunction or thrombocytopenia.
        iii. Vascular disorder.

N.B.
    a. Always take a *fresh* blood sample with a new plastic syringe.
    b. Cause minimal tissue trauma, or extravascular clotting factors may be stimulated, interfering with tests.
    c. Advisable to take *control* samples from *normal* dogs at the same time.

Tests

1. Clotting time

A rather crude but useful test for practice:
    a. Take 1–2 ml blood into a plain glass test-tube or plain plastic tube. Keep warm (*c.* 37 °C) and gently oscillate until strands of fibrin are seen:
        i. Normal time: 4–10 min.
        ii. Time >10 min: clotting defect (not platelet or vascular).
        iii. Time <4 min: possible tissue trauma in sampling?
or
    b. Use a capillary (microhaematocrit) tube, and fill with blood. Break the tube every 30 sec until strands of fibrin are found. Normal clotting time: 3–4 min.

2. Clot retraction

    Leave 5 ml of clotted blood to stand at room temperature.
    Normally: the clot retracts within a few hours.
    Slow retraction: lack of fibrinogen? Thrombocytopenia or platelet dysfunction?

3. Bleeding time

    a. Use a lancet or fine scalpel blade, nick a hairless area of skin (pinna).
    b. Gently stroke or blot with cotton wool or filter paper until bleeding ceases.
    Normal time: <5 min.
    Prolonged bleeding: platelet or vascular disorder (or DIC)?

4. Platelet count

    a. Collect sample in an EDTA bottle.
    b. Count with a conventional haemocytometer
        Normal: 150 000–500 000/mm^3.
        <30 000: significant thrombocytopenia.

Other tests (mainly by specialised laboratories)

1. Prothrombin time (assesses extravascular clotting factors)
   a. Collect 2·5 ml fresh blood into an oxalate or citrate tube.
   b. Incubate 0·1 ml plasma with Simplastin (Warner).
   c. Assess clotting time in plasma, together with control sample.
      Normal: <12 sec (pups <30 sec).
      Prolonged in Warfarin poisoning, hepatic failure,
      hypovitaminosis K, Factor VII or X deficiency, disseminated
      intravascular coagulation (DIC).

2. Activated partial thromboplastin time (assesses intravascular
factors) (specialist laboratory test for which very fresh blood is
required)
Normal result: 14–25 sec.
Prolonged in persistent Warfarin poisoning, DIC, Factor VIII deficiency
(true haemophilia), Factor IX, X, XI or XII deficiency, Von
Willebrand disease.

3. Fibrin degradation products
(specialist laboratory test—serum required)
Elevated in disseminated intravascular coagulation (DIC).

4. Specific clotting factor tests
For congenital clotting defects or platelet dysfunction.
Specialist assessments, not generally available.

Treatment
   a. Warfarin poisoning and hepatic failure
      Require Vitamin K₁ for at least 4 days (p. 246).
   b. Many platelet disorders respond to corticosteroid therapy.
   c. Local bleeding may be stemmed with pressure.
   d. Many haemorrhagic disorders may be relieved with transfusion
      of *fresh* blood: platelets and clotting factors do not survive
      storage well (p. 252).
   e. Dogs with congenital coagulation disorders:
      i. Should be protected against trauma, as far as possible.
      ii. Relatives should be carefully screened for clotting.
      iii. Specific clotting factors are not available for dogs.

REFERENCES AND FURTHER READING

Couto C. G. (1982) Therapy for abnormal erythropoiesis. *J. Am. Vet. Med. Assoc.* **181**,
   501.

Crispin S. M. (1981) Practical aspects of fluid and blood administration. *Proc. Assoc. Vet. Anaes. G.B.* **9**, 86.
Dodds J. (1983) Inherited coagulation disorders in the dog. *In Pract.* **5**, 54.
Dorner J. L. (1974) Normal prothrombin time and partial thromboplastin times of the dog. *J. Am. Anim. Hosp. Assoc.* **10**, 412.
Evans R. J., Jones D. R. E. and Gruffydd-Jones T. J. (1982) Esential thrombocythaemia in the dog and cat: a report of four cases. *J. Small Anim. Pract.* **23**, 457.
Feldman B. F. (1981) Coagulopathies *J. Am. Vet. Med. Assoc.* **179**, 555.
Feldman B. F. (1983) Management of the Anemic dog. In: Kirk R. W. (ed.) *Current Veterinary Therapy.* VIII. Philadelphia, Saunders.
Greene C. E. (1975) Disseminated intravascular coagulation in the dog: a review. *J. Am. Anim. Hosp. Assoc.* **11**, 674.
Harvey J. W. (1980) Canine hemolytic anemias. *J. Am. Vet. Med. Assoc.* **176**, 970.
Harvey J. W., French T. W. and Meyer D. J. (1982) Iron deficiency anemia in dogs. *J. Am. Anim. Hosp. Assoc.* **18**, 946.
Johnessee J. A. and Hurvitz A. I. (1983) Thrombocytopenia. In: Kirk R. W. (ed.) *Current Veterinary Therapy* VIII. Philadelphia, Saunders.
Kociba G. J. (1976) The diagnosis of hemostatic disorders. *Vet. Clin. N. Am.* **6**,(4), 609.
Matus R. E., Leifer C. E. and McEwen E. G. (1983) Acute lymphoblastic leukemia in the dog: a review of 30 cases. *J. Am. Vet. Med. Assoc.* **183**, 859.
Morgan R. V. (1982) Blood dyscrasias with testicular tumors in dogs. *J. Am. Anim. Hosp. Assoc.* **18**, 970.
O'Rourke L. G. (1983) Practical blood transfusions. In: Kirk R. W. (ed.) *Current Veterinary Therapy* VIII. Philadelphia, Saunders.
Owen R ap R. and Glen J. B. (1972) Factors to be considered when making canine blood and blood products available for transfusion. *Vet. Rec.* **91**, 406.
Penny R. H. C. and Carlisle C. H. (1970) The bone marrow of the dog: a comparative study of biopsy material obtained from the iliac crest, rib and sternum. *J. Small Anim. Pract.* **11**, 727.
Perman V., Osborne C. A. and Stevens J. B. (1974) Bone marrow biopsy. *Vet. Clin. N. Am.* **4**,(2), 293.
Pichler M. E. and Turnwald G. H. (1985) Blood transfusion in the dog and cat I. *Comp. Cont. Pract. Ed. Vet.* **7**, 64 & 115.
Rebar A. H. and Boon G. D. (1981) An approach to the diagnosis of bleeding disorders in the dog. *J. Am. Anim. Hosp. Assoc.* **17**, 227.
Ruehl W. (1982) Rational therapy in disseminated intravascular coagulation. *J. Am. Vet. Med. Assoc.* **181**, 76.
Schalm O. W., Jain J. C. and Carroll E. J. (1975) *Veterinary Hematology,* 3rd ed. Philadelphia, Lea & Febiger.
Searcy G. P. (1976) The differential diagnosis of anemia. *Vet. Clin. N. Am.* **6**(4), 567.
Sherding R. G., Wilson G. P. and Kociba G. J. (1981) Bone marrow hypoplasia in eight dogs with Sertoli cell tumour. *J. Am. Vet. Med. Assoc.* **178**, 497.
Weiser M. G. (1981) Correlative approach to anemia in dogs and cats. *J. Am. Anim. Hosp. Assoc.* **17**, 286.

Chapter 43

Acute Poisoning

Innumerable potential poisons exist in the modern environment. When a call concerning suspected poisoning is made to a practice, the following points should be borne in mind.

A. CLIENTS' ATTITUDES

1. Often there are feelings of guilt
   —therefore the history may be unreliable.
2. Fear of the worst causes anger and panic.
3. Tend to blame *any* acute illness on poisoning.
4. Look for recriminations and scapegoats.
5. Often blame neighbours, though uncommonly involved.

B. GENERAL PRINCIPLES

1. In *suspected* poisoning, proof may be very difficult.
2. Specific antidotes are *not* available for most poisons.
3. *Symptomatic* treatment and support are important.
4. Be seen to be acting with urgency and without panic.
5. *Record* all possible details carefully.

COMMON POISONS AND MAJOR SIGNS

1. *Warfarin* (coumarins) → multiple haemorrhages;
   weakness or collapse and anaemia.
2. *Alphachloralose* (rodenticide) → hyperexcitability, then depression; hypothermia in small dogs.

3. *Metaldehyde* (slug bait) → incoordination, apprehension, depression, salivation, muscle tremors, tachypnoea, hyperaesthesia, convulsions, nystagmus.
4. *Organophosphates* (insecticides and molluscicides) → cholinergic stimulation: ataxia, muscle twitching, dyspnoea, 'cyanosis', salivation, diarrhoea, abdominal pain, urination, miosis, bradydysrhythmias.
5. *Paraquat* (herbicide) → vomiting, anorexia, oral ulceration → better, then progressive *dyspnoea*, severe cyanosis and air hunger.
6. *Glycol* (antifreeze) → CNS depression, disorientation → seizures and coma, acute renal failure (*see* p. 163), tachypnoea, cyanosis.
7. *Strychnine* (mole poison): apprehension, restlessness → tetanic convulsions—with any stimulation.
8. *Lead* (old paint, old batteries): *vague* signs—slight tremors → convulsions, blindness, gastrointestinal upset and abdominal *pain,* anorexia, listlessness.
9. *Chlorinated hydrocarbons* (insecticides) cause: hyperaesthesia, tremors, convulsions.
10. *Others:*
    a. Drugs for human use: aspirin, sedatives, contraceptives, laxatives.
    b. Household chemicals: disinfectants, bleach.
    c. House and garden plants: laburnum sticks, oleander, wood chippings (yew, redwood).
    d. Carbon monoxide: malfunctioning boilers, fires.
    e. Fertilizers.
    f. Weedkillers (sodium chlorate; 2,4,5-T).
    g. Many other forms of rubbish (dogs are *scavengers*).

DIFFERENTIAL DIAGNOSIS OF ACUTE DISORDERS
resembling 'poisonings'

1. Road accident or other trauma.
2. Infectious canine hepatitis.
3. Parvovirus infection.
4. Haemorrhagic gastroenteritis (HGE) (Chapter 20).
5. Eclampsia and other calcium disturbances (Chapter 36).
6. Heat stroke/hypothermia.
7. Snake bites.
8. Interstitial (viral) pneumonia (Chapter 2).
9. Acute cardiac decompensation (Chapter 9).
10. Hypoadrenocorticalism (Addisonian crisis) (Chapter 36).
11. Other acute abdominal disorders (Chapter 20).
12. Primary epilepsy.

APPROACH TO SUSPECTED POISONING

History (questions to be posed over the telephone):
   a. Access—does the dog stray—any known poisons available?
   b. Speed of onset and course of signs.
   c. General recent health of animal.
   d. Major symptoms?
       i. Neurological (convulsions or depression).
       ii. Gastrointestinal.
       iii. Respiratory.
       iv. Haemorrhage.

Immediate action (by client?) especially if the poison is known:
   a. Prevent further access.
   b. Identify the poison (drug or chemical).
   c. Induce vomiting?:
       Not for phenolics, petroleum derivatives, corrosives;
       not if convulsing or already distressed.
       i. Dose with a crystal of washing soda (Na_2CO_3).
       ii. Mustard on the tongue?
       iii. 1 teaspoonful of hydrogen peroxide?
       iv. Apomorphine s.c. (0–1 mg/kg body weight).
           But very violent and usually *unnecessary*.
           And keep a sample of vomitus for analysis? (expensive).
   d. Remove all trace of the substance from dog's skin and coat:
       i. Warm water and soft soap or detergent.
       ii. Ether/turpentine/Swarfega—if solvents are needed.
       iii. *Then wash off.*
       iv. Dry and warm the animal.
   e. Give milk/water/egg white to drink.

Findings

Be brief, but careful, over the clinical examination:
   a. Tremors/convulsions/depression/coma?
   b. Mucous membranes—pale/congested/cyanosed?
                        —ulcerated/inflamed (caustics).
   c. Respirations—rate/character/depth?
   d. Rectal temperature, heart rate?
   e. Gastrointestinal signs?
   f. Any evidence of *trauma*/other circumstances?
   g. Contamination of coat/skin?
   h. Haemorrhages?
Record all findings

Further management—take *care* in handling a dog with convulsions

   a. Consider gastrointestinal lavage if within 2 hours:
       i. Alternate washing soda with milk drink or saline.
      ii. Wash out the stomach with warm saline (5–10 ml/kg).
     iii. Via a stomach tube under general anaesthesia?
      iv. Administer sodium sulphate (60 mg/kg) orally,
          —as a mild purgative.
   b. Consider absorbants—via stomach tube.
       i. Activated charcoal (as a slurry).
      ii. Bismuth/kaolin.
   c. Consider whether there is a known *antidote* e.g.:
       i. Warfarin—Vitamin K_1 (Konakion; Searle) 2 mg/kg i.m.
          b.i.d.—may need to be repeated daily for up to 10 days
          with modern anticoagulants.
      ii. Paraquat—Fuller's Earth or clay orally (stomach
          tube); only effective if given *immediately* after
          ingestion.
     iii. Organophosphates
          Atropine (0·25 mg/kg s.c.).
          Pralidoxime (Protopam; Ayerst) 20 mg/kg i.m. b.i.d.
          Produce partial relief of effects.
      iv. Glycol—ethyl alcohol 5 ml/kg of 20 per cent
          —then 10 per cent glucose i.v.
          Effective if given soon after ingestion. Repeat 6 hourly.
       v. Strychnine:
          Glyceryl guaiacolate 100 mg/kg of 1 per cent i.v.
          Diazepam (Valium; Roche) or barbiturate i.v.
      vi. Lead—calcium disodium versonate (maximum of 75 mg/
          kg/day of 10 per cent i.v. for 5 days).
     vii. Sodium chlorate—methylene blue 2 ml/kg of 1 per cent
          i.v.

Supportive treatment—very important

   a. Maintain the *airway*—oxygen needed (Chapter 1)?
   b. Provide *warmth* if not hyperthermic and check temperature.
   c. Intravenous fluid therapy:
       i. Normal saline (50 mg/kg body weight over 2 hours).
      ii. Glucose 5 per cent (20 ml/kg if no urine produced).
     iii. Calcium gluconate 10 per cent (10–50 ml).
   d. Sedation if convulsing or hyperaesthetic?;
       i. Diazepam (valium; Roche) (0·3 mg/kg i.v.).
      ii. Pentobarbitone sodium (10–30 mg/kg i.v. or i.p.).
     iii. General anaesthesia.

If the animal dies or euthanasia is required

   a. Make notes of all findngs (normal and abnormal).

   b. Retain a sample of gastric contents.

   c. Retain samples of liver, kidney, blood and urine (fresh and in alcohol/formol saline).

   d. Find an analyst—analysis is only of value if known substances are being assessed, and it is very expensive.

FURTHER READING

Clarke M. L. (1984) Poisoning. In: Chandler E. A. et al. (ed.), *Canine Medicine and Therapeutics*, 2nd Ed. Oxford, Blackwell Scientific.

Oehme F. W. (1983) Chemical and Physical Disorders. In: Kirk R. W. (ed.), *Current Veterinary Therapy* VIII Philadelphia, Saunders.

Index

abdomen, bloated, 194
  'dropped', 194, 213
abdominal auscultation, 122
  cyst, 195, 227
  discomfort, 106, 126, 180
  disorders, acute, 121–24, 164, 196,
    258
  distension, 192–95, 197
  effusions, 192
  enlargement, 60, 61, 147, 192–95, 206,
    213, 228
  investigation, 194
  fluoroscopy, 201
  haemorrhage, 192
  mass, 62, 161, 172, 190, 197, 217,
    227
    differential diagnosis, 193
    radiology, 197
  neoplasia, 111, 192, 194, 217, 227
  pain, 106, 107, 121, 122, 125, 132,
    145, 157, 159, 160, 164, 172, 178,
    180, 190, 216, 228, 258
  palpation, 117, 122, 126, 132, 137,
    171, 172, 174, 180, 183, 190,
    194, 225
  paracentesis, 92, 195
    in acute disorders, 122
    in pancreatitis, 160
  peristalsis, 122
  radiography, 196–202
  trauma, 126, 192, 197
  tympany, 194
abscess, foreign body, 16, 241
  mediastinal, 18
  pharyngeal, 1, 241
  prostatic, 177
  pulmonary, 13
absorbants, alimentary, 141, 260
acetylpromazine, 115, 151, 152
acid-base disturbances, 54, 99, 106, 121
acidosis, in diabetes mellitus, 53, 220
  in dysrhythmias, 72
  effect on the heart, 54, 99
acromegaly, 206, 220, 226, 229, 235
ACTH level, 215, 216
  stimulation test, 214, (Fig. 12) 216
'acute abdomen', see Abdominal
    disorders, acute
Addison's disease, see
    Hypoadrenocorticalism
adenovirus, 5, 12, 145

ADH, 205
  response test, 231
adhesion, following trauma, 193
  intestinal, 125
adrenal disorders, 212–17
  insufficiency, see
    Hypoadrenocorticalism
  neoplasia, 212, 215, 216, 217
adrenalectomy, 215
β-adrenergic blockade, 75, 92
  for atrial fibrillation, 73
  for hypoglycaemia, 222
  for tachycardia, 73
  production from phaeochromocytoma,
    217
  stimulants, 4, 73, 100
adrenocortical atrophy, 216
  hyperplasia, 212
  neoplasia, 212, 215, 217
adrenocorticotrophic hormone, see ACTH
aerophagia, 102, 105, 112
Afghans, 206, 234
aggression, 225
air hunger, 30, 59, 258
airway foreign body, 1, 4, 16, 27, 30
  infections, 5, 10
  inflammation, 5
    diagnosis, 6
    treatment, 6
  neoplasia, 1, 3, 26
  obstruction, 1, 22, 26, 28, 53, 54, 65
    brachycephalic, 1
    diagnosis, 3 -
    effect on heart, 70
    surgery, 4
    penetration, 16, 17
    radiography, 33
    radiology, 3, 34, 36
    trauma, 1, 4, 22
alactasia, 127
albumin level, low, see
    Hypoalbuminaemia
aldosterone, in cardiac failure, 57
alimentary foreign body, location, 197
  penetration, 192
  infections, 105, 126, 131
  obstruction, 125
  radiology for obstruction, 197
  radiology, 118, 196–9
  tract (rupture), 192
  see also Gastric; Intestinal disorders

alkaline phosphatase, 147, **149**, 156, 212, 213
see also Liver enzyme levels
alopecia, 204, 207, 213, 226
differential diagnosis, **215**
Alsations, see German shepherds
ALT level, 145, **149**
aluminium hydroxide, 103, 106, 108, 123, 142, 167, 212
alveolar disorders, **10**
radiology, **35**
see also Pulmonary disorders
ammonia level, see Hyperammonaemia
ammonia tolerance test, 151
amylase level, in pancreatitis, 122, 160
amyloidosis, 13, 147, 153, 158, 165, 167
anabolic steroids,
  for anaemia, 248, 252
  for hepatic failure, 152
  for renal failure, 167, 168
anaemia, 65, 108, 165, **245–56**
  autoimmune haemolytic, 155, **236**, 248
  chronic, 246, 247, 248
  differential diagnosis, **245**
  haemolytic, 155, **248**, 249
  haemorrhagic, 245, 249
  hypoplastic, 246, 247, 248, 249, 250
  in hypothyroidism, 207
  investigation of, **249**
  isoimmune haemolytic, 248
  in puppies, 248
  regenerative, 237, 246, 248, **250**
  traumatic, 245
  treatment, **251**
  types of, **249**
anaerobes, pleural, 16, 19
anaesthesia,
  for airway obstruction, 3
  for bronchoscopy, 39
  for endoscopy, 117
  effect on heart, 51, 54, **58**, 62, 99
  in liver disease, 153
anaesthetic gases, in cardiac arrest, 100
  hypoxia, 58
anal foreign body, 189
  lesions
    and constipation, 189
    and hypercalcaemia, 211
  sac abscess, 189
  stricture, 189
  see also Perianal fistulae
analgesia, 24, 122, 160, 212
  see also opiates
anaphylaxis, 62
anastomoses, see Shunts

androgens, for false pregnancy,226
  in prostatic disease, 177
angiography, cardiac, 37, 48, **85**
  in cyanosis, 68
  portal, 148, **201**
Angiostrongylus vasorum, 12, 13, 37, 39, 246
angiotensin
  antagonist, 94
  in cardiac failure, 57
anisocytosis in anaemia, 250
anoestrus, 207, 213, 226
  see also Oestrus, abnormal
antemetic, central, 123
  gastric, 108, 123
anthelmintics, 6, 14, **128–9**
antibiotics,
  in airway disorders, 7, 8
  not antipyretics, 241
  in endocarditis, 50
  in hepatic failure, 152
  in intestinal disorders, 126, 132, 142
  for myocarditis, 52
  persistent use of, 136, 142
  for prostatic infections, 178, 180
  in pulmonary disorders, 14
  for pyothorax, 19
  in pyrexia, 243
  for urinary infections, **171**
antidiuretic hormone, see ADH
antidotes for poisoning, **260**
antihistamines for coughing, 7
antinuclear antibody test, 239
antipyretics, 237, 244
ANTU poisoning, 10
aortic body tumour, 18
  outflow obstruction, 58
  (persistent right aortic arch), 46, 102
  stenosis, 46, 58, 63, 88
  surgery, 92
apexcardiography, 79, 89
appetite, diminished—see inappetance
  increased—see polyphagia
arrhythmia, sinus, **70**
  'tumultuous heart', 73
  see also Dysrhythmias, cardiac
arteriolar dilation—see vasodilation
arteriosclerosis, coronary, 50, 51
arteriovenous fistulae, 65
  see also Shunts
artificial pacemaker, **74**
  respiration, 3
ascarid infection, 12, 128

ascites, 17, 46, 52, 60, 144, 145, 147,
    167, 175, 227
  differential diagnosis, 192–3
  investigation, 194
  radiography, 197
  treatment, 93, 195
aspirin—see salicylates
AST, 149
  see also Liver enzymes
asthma, see Bronchospasm
ataxia, 63, 65, 210, 221, 258
atherosclerosis, coronary, 51
atrial dilatation, 50, 84, 85
  ectopic (premature) beats, 72
  fibrillation, 73, 75
  therapy, 73, 95
  flutter, 73, 75
  septal defects, 45, 88
  tachycardias, paroxysmal, 73
atrioventricular block, 72, 74
atropine, 4, 71, 72, 74, 123, 133, 160, 260
auscultation, abdominal, 122
  in cardiac failure, 59
  of cardiac sounds, 32, 79–82
  in dysrhythmias, 71–3
  in pleural disorders, 17, 19
  respiratory, 6, 11, 17, 32
  thoracic, 32
  see also Murmurs, cardiac
autoimmune disease, 164, 167, 216,
    236–40
  haemolytic anaemia, 155, 236, 248
  pericarditis, 52
  polyarteritis, 239, 242
  in pyrexia, 242
  thrombocytopenia, 237
'autotransfusion', 20
axis deviation, right, 48

babesiasis, 156, 248
bacterial overgrowth, intestinal, 127, 134,
    135, 136, 140
bacteriology,
  in endocarditis, 50
  faecal, 138
  in peritonitis, 195
  in pyrexia, 243
  respiratory, 3, 6, 37, 41
  urinary, 171, 173, 184
barium enema, 132, 141, 191, 199
  meal, 108, 123, 129, 132, 198
  swallow, 37, 118
barking, 5

'barrel chest', 31
Basenjis, 248
Beagles, 46
beats, 'missed' or 'dropped', 72
  premature or ectopic, 72
  see also Dysrhythmias
behaviour in false pregnancy, 225
  hypersexed, 217
behavioural disorders, 141
  diarrhoea, 136, 141
  incontinence, 186
  see also Psychological and psychogenic
    disorders
beta blockade, see β-adrenergic blockade
bicarbonate, 72, 100, 106, 123, 142, 160,
    162, 174, 220
bile duct obstruction, 146, 149, 150, 156,
    159
  rupture, 145, 192, 193
bilirubin, 146, 147, 150, 155–6
biopsy, bone marrow, 243, 251
  colonic, 141
  gastric, 108, 119
  hepatic, 146, 148, 150, 151
  intestinal, 140
  lung, 12, 42
  lymph node, 243
  parathyroid, 210, 212
  prostatic, 180
  renal, 164, 166, 168, 239
  for thoracic lesions, 19, 42
  thyroid, 208, 210
  see also Cytology
biurate crystals, in urine, 151, 172
bladder, absence of, 170, 199
  atony, 193
    treatment, 187
  calculi, 172, 189, 199, 200
  displacement, 185, 190
  immature, 170, 185, 200
  infections, 170
  neck lesions, 185
  neoplasia, 172, 174, 182, 185, 190,
    199, 200, 246
  radiology, 171, 173, 174, 196, 197,
    199, 200
  retroflexed, 172
  ruptured, 175, 193, 199, 200
  sphincter congenital dysfunction,
    170
    incoordination, 185, 186
  see also Cystitis; Urinary disorders
bleeding disorders, 238, 245, 252
  time, 238, 254
blindness, 258

blood, 'autotransfusion', 20
  bacterial culture, 50, **243**
  in faeces, **133**, 136, **247**
  gas analysis, 48, 68, **88**, 89
  levels, *see under* individual constituent
  pressure recordings, 48, 79, **88**
  sampling fresh, 254
  transfusions, 237, 246, **252**
  cross-matching, 252
  incompatible, 155, 248, 252
'blue eye', 145
borborygmi, 126, 136
Border collies, 46, 247
Bordetella bronchiseptica, 5
botulism, 66, 114
Boxers, 2, 29, 46, 51, 107, 117, 206, 209, 221
brachycephalic breeds, 1, 4, 29, 55, 65, 71
  airway obstruction, 1, 4, 28, 29
bradycardia, 54, 63, 71, **72**
  in hyperparathyroidism, 211
  in hypoadrenocorticalism, 216
  in hypothyroidism, 207
bradydysrhythmias, 55, **71**, 258
  therapy, **74**
breeds, giant, 50, 73
  large, and cardiomyopathy, 50
  and endocarditis, 49
  and hypercalcitonism, 210
  and incontinence, 185
  and pericardial haemorrhage, 52
  see under individual breed
bromsulphthalein (BSP) retention test, 150
bronchial obstruction, **1–2**, 10, 32
bronchial washings, 6
bronchiectasis, 5
  radiology, 36
  treatment, 7
bronchitis, 2, 5, 11
  radiology, 36
  treatment, 7
bronchodilatation, **4**, 7, 8, 92, 96
bronchofibrescopes, 38
bronchograms, air, 36
bronchography, 3, 6, **37**
bronchopneumonia, 5, 6, **10**, 13, 25, 31, 241
  radiology, 36
  treatment, **14**
bronchoscopy, 3, 6, 28, **37–9**
bronchospasm, 2, 5
brucellosis, 241
bruising, *see* Purpura
bullae, lung, 12, 17
  ruptured, 12
Bulldogs, English, 2, 46

Cairns, 172
calcinosis cutis, 213
calcium disturbances, 54, 66, 210, 212, 258
campylobacter infection, 131, 133, 135
capillary hydrostatic pressure, raised, 16
  permeability, increased, 10, 17
  refill, slow, 62, 99, 216
  see also Shock
captopril, 91, **95**
carcinoma—*see* neoplasia
cardiac arrest, 53, 54, 72, 74, **99–101**
  auscultation, *see* Auscultation, cardiac
  bypass, 92
  catheterization, 48, 68, 85, **88**
  chamber enlargement, 57, **84**
  conduction disturbances, 50, 72
  congenital lesions, **45–8**
  decompensation, **57**, 59, 60, 258
    acute, 58, 96
  diagnosis, *see* Apexcardiography;
    Auscultation; Electrocardiography;
    Phonocardiography
  dilatation, 80
  disease, investigation, **77–90**
  disorders, acquired, **49**
    congenital, **45**
  dysrhythmias, *see* Dysrhythmias,
    cardiac
  enlargement, audible, 32
    in cardiac failure, 59
    in congenital disorders, 48
    in cor pulmonale, 53
    in hyperthyroidism, 209
    obstructing the airway, 2, 18, 26
    pericardial, 52
    radiography for, **83–6**
  failure, **57–64**
    acute, 59
    treatment for, **96**
    chronic, left-sided, 58
    compensation for, **57**
    congestive, 16, 45, 51, **61**, 64, 135, 148, 192
    diuresis for, **93**
    and polydipsia, **230**
    radiographic signs, **84**
  investigation, **77–82**
  left-sided, 46, 49, **58–60**, 63
  management, **91–8**
  radiographic signs, **84**
  right-sided, 16, 46, 49, 52, 53, **60–61**, 64, 148
  functional disturbances, 55, 63

cardiac arrest, (*cont.*)
  glycosides, *see* Glycosides, cardiac
  hypertrophy, 57
  imaging, 90
  insufficiency, 51, 53, **63**, 65
  lesions, **45–52**
  massage, 100
  monitors, 101
  murmurs, *see* Murmurs, cardiac
  neoplasia, 51, 62
  output, loss, 51, **63**, 74
  radiography, 60, 61, 62, **83–6**
  rate, 32, 79
    fast, 70, 73
    slow, 72
  resuscitation, **99–101**
  rhythm, **70–6**
    escape, 73
    gallop, 59, **80**
    variable, 73
  shunts, left-to-right, 45, 61
    right-to-left, 45, 68
  size, normal, 83
  sounds, *see* Sounds, cardiac
  tamponade, 52, 58, 61
  trauma, 22, 50, 52, 88
  treatment, 74–6, **91–8**
  valves, *see* Valvular
  see also Myocardial and pericardial
    disorders
cardiogenic shock, *see* Shock
cardiomyopathy, 57, 58, 60, 62
  hypertrophic, 62
  idiopathic, 50, 60, 62, 92
castration for prostatic disorders, 177, 179,
  180
cataract, 218
catecholamines, 55
  in dysrhythmias, 72
  excess activity, 99, 217
  see also β-adrenergic
catheterization
  see Cardiac catheterization
  see Urinary catheterization
caudal vena cava, enlargement, 84
  obstruction, 62, 64
Cavalier King Charles Spaniel, 49
central venous pressure, 88, 123
cerebral hypoxia, 63, 65
chemodectomy, *see* heart base tumour
Chihuahuas, 46, 49
cholecystography, 148, 151, **201**
cholestasis, 146, 150
cholesterol level, 151, 168, 207, 213,
  219

chordae tendineae, 49
  rupture, 58
chylothorax, **16**, 22, **41**
  therapy, **20**
chylous effusion, **16**, **193**
  pseudochylous effusion, 16
cimetidine, 103, 108, 142, 167
circulating volume, 57, 83
circulatory overload, 57
  treatment, **91**
clot retraction, 238, **254**
clotting factors, assessment, **254–5**
  disturbed, 144, 147, 151, 245
  times, 147, **254**
CNS congenital lesions, 66, 186
  depression, 258
  disturbances, **65–6**, 112, 147, 186, 222
    in dyspnoea, 27
  haemorrhage, 66
  hypoxia, 65
  and incontinence, 186
  irritation, 112
  lesions, 65–6, 112, 186, 222
  metabolic disorders, affecting, **65–6**, 147
  neoplasia, 66, 186, 222, 241
  trauma, 10, 23, 66, 186, 241
  and vomiting, 111–12
  see also Convulsions: Seizures
coagulation disorders, **245**
  and the abdomen, 192
  and the alimentary tract, 133
  in hepatic failure, 144, 147
  intravascular, *see* Disseminated
    intravascular coagulation
  in respiratory disease, 10, 14, 16
  tests, *see* Clotting
  and urinary tract, 183
coccidia, 129, 131, 133
Cocker spaniels, 165, 218
cold, intolerance to, 207
collagen disorders, 236
collapse, 47, 51, 63, **65–9**, 71, 99, 160,
  221
  diagnostic procedure, **67**
  differential diagnosis, **65**
  in haemorrhage, 246
  laboratory tests, 68
Collies, 159
colitis, **131**, 132, 133, 135
  and tenesmus, 189
  therapy, 132
colon, irritable, 132, 133
colonic biopsy, 141
  disorders, **131–3**, 137, 189, 199
    treatment, **132**

colonic biopsy, (cont.)
  foreign bodies, 131, 133, 135, 137, 189,
    199
  neoplasia, 131, 133, 135, 137, 189, 199
  obstruction, 131, 199
  radiology, 141, 196, **199**
  surgery, 123
comedones, 207, 213
conduction disturbances, 50, 72
congenital aortic stenosis, 46
  cardiac defects, surgical correction, **92**
  lesions, **45-8**, 204
  cardiovascular anomalies, 46
  CNS lesions, 66, 186
  haemolysis, 155, 248
  haemophilia, 245, 255
  hypopituitarism, 203
  mitral dysplasia, 46, 58
  portosystemic shunts, **146**, 151, 201
  pulmonic stenosis, 46
  renal dysplasia, 165, 204
  shunts, **45**, 204
  spinal lesions, 186
  tracheal hypoplasia, 2
  tricuspid dysplasia, 46, 60
  urinary lesions, **170**
congestive cardiac failure, see Cardiac
    failure, congestive
constipation, **131**, 177, 179, **189**, 207
  treatment, 133
contrast media, radiographic, see
    Angiography; Barium;
    Bronchography;
    Cholecystography;
    Pneumocystography;   Urography;
    Vagino-urethography
contusions, 22
convulsions, 166, 210, 220, 258
  see also' Seizure
Coombs' test, 237, 239, 251
copper toxicosis, 147
coprophagy, 136, 159
Corgis, 172
corneal lipidosis, 207, 213
coronary arteriosclerosis, 50, 51
coronavirus, 105
cor pulmonale, 7, **53**, 60
corticosteroids,
  in acute abdominal disorders, 123
  in airway disorders, 4, 7
  in anaemia, 246, 248, 251, 255
  in autoimmune disease, 168, 237, 243,
    248
  in chronic diarrhoea (malabsorption),
    141

corticosteroids, (cont.)
  excess administration, 108, 212, 230
  in hepatic disease, 152
  in hypoadrenocorticalism, 217
  in myocarditis, 52
  in pancreatitis, 160
  in persistent diarrhoea, 141
  sudden withdrawal, 216
cortisol level, 214, 216
coughing, **25**, 65, 112
  in airway irritation, 5
  in airway obstruction, 2
  in cardiac failure, 46, **59**, 61
  differential diagnosis, **27**
  productive, 7, 11
  in pulmonary disorders, 11
  therapy, **7**
  in thoracic trauma, 23
  unproductive, 7, 12
coumarins, see Poisoning, warfarin
cramp, 210
craniomandibular osteopathy, 114
creatinine level, 166
crepitations, respiratory, 32
cretinism, 206
cricopharyngeal achalasia, 102, 103, 113
culture, bacterial, see Bacteriology
Cushing's syndrome, see
    Hyperadrenocorticalism
cyanosis, cardiac, 47, 59, 63, 99
  differential diagnosis, **68**
  in poisoning, 258
  respiratory, 2, 11, 12, 13, 17, 23, 26
    30
cystic, see Bladder
cystitis, **170**, 182, 189
  emphysematous, 175
  haemorrhagic, 175
cystography, 184, **200**
cytology, for serous effusions, 40, **41**, 195
  tracheal, 3, 6, 38, **39**
  urinary, 174, 179

Dachshunds, 49, 172, 213, 218
Dalmations, 172
decompensation, cardiac, 57, 59
  renal, 165
defaecation, frequency, 132
  see also Faeces
defibrillation, cardiac, 73, 100
dehydration, 106, 121, 123, 164, 165, 205
    211, 216, 228
dental sepsis, 241

dexamethasone suppression test, 214
diabetes insipidus, **205**, 229
mellitus, 149, 153, 175, 215, **217–21**,
229
diabetic ketoacidosis, 53, 218, 220
dialysis, peritoneal, 164
diaphragm, pressure, 26
ruptured, 17, 18, 22, 35
repair, 20
diarrhoea, 121, 126, **127**
acute haemorrhagic, differential
diagnosis, **133**
chronic, **134–43**
pathogenesis, **134**
persistent, differential diagnosis,
134
investigation, **136**
management, **141**
psychological, 136
and weight loss, 233
with blood, 132, **133**
with mucus, 132
DIC, *see* Disseminated intravascular
coagulation
diet, in anaemia, 248, 251
bland, 106, 137, 141
inadequate, 233
inappropriate, in diarrhoea, 134
in obesity, 235
polydipsia and, 230
quality, poor, 233
salt-free, 94, 152, 168
and urinary calculi, **174**
weight loss and, **233**
dietary excess, 134
in diarrhoea, **134**
intolerance, 134
management in alimentary disorders,
137, 141
cardiac failure, 94
chylothorax, 20
diabetes mellitus, 220
hepatic failure, 152
nephrotic syndrome, 168
renal failure, 166, 168
digitalization, **94–5**
for atrial fibrillation, 73
see also Glycosides, cardiac
digoxin, *see* Glycosides, cardiac
Dipylidium caninum, 128
Dirofilaria imitis, 12, 13, 37
dirofilariasis, 53, 60
disaccharidase insufficiency, 127, 135
disc, prolapsed intervertebral, 66, 186
disopyramide, 73, **75**

disseminated intravascular coagulation,
160, 245
diagnosis, 255
distemper, 5, 12, 105, 113, 239
diuresis, 14, 153, 230
for congestive cardiac failure, **93**, 96
for diabetes insipidus, 205
for false pregnancy, 226
iatrogenic, 230
intravenous, 96
in renal failure, 164, 168
osmotic, 164, 218
dosing, careless, 10
oral misdosing, 2
drowning, 10
drug toxicity, effect on the heart, 51
ductus arteriosus, patent, *see* Patent
ductus arteriosus
duodenal fluid sample, 140
duodenal
gastric reflux, 110, 111
obstruction, 105
ulcer, 129
dwarfism, 203, 204
dyschezia, 189
dysphagia, 2, 102, 233
differential diagnosis, **114**
dysphonia, 2, 6, 26, 209
dyspnoea,
in airway obstruction, 2
in cardiac failure, 45, 59, 60, 61
differential diagnosis of, **25–7**
pleural, 17, 18
in poisoning, 258
pulmonary, 11, 12
in pyrexia, 242
in thoracic trauma, 22
in thyroid neoplasia, 209
dysrhythmias, cardiac, 23, 51, **70–3**, 106,
242, 258
acute, 62, 63
diagnosis, 74
therapy for, **74–6**
gastric dysrhythmia, 105
see also Bradydysrhythmias;
Tachydysrhythmias
dystocia, 190
dysuria, 172, 174, 177, 178, **189**, 197

E.C.G.—*see* electrocardiography
Echinococcus granulosus, 128
echocardiography, 49, 89
eclampsia, 27, 54, 66, 210, 258

ectopic beats, 72
effusions, abdominal, **192–3**
  neoplastic, 16–18, 41–2
  pericardial, **52**
  pleural, **16–18**, 26, **40–2**, 243
  and polydipsia, 230
  purulent, 16, **41, 192**
  transudative, 16, 17, **41, 192–3**
electrical alternans, 52
electrocardiography, **86**
  artefacts, 86
  in endocarditis, 50
  in heart blocks, 72
  in hypoadrenocorticalism, 216
  in metabolic disturbances, **53–4**
  in tachydysrhythmias, **73**
  voltages reduced, 52
  waveforms, 72, 86
  see also P wave; QRS complex;
    T wave
electrolyte disturbances and ECGs, 54
  and the heart, 51, **53–4**
embolism, pulmonary, 13
  septic, 51
emergency,
  abdominal, **121–4**
  cardiac, **99–101**
  poisonings, **257–61**
  respiratory, 3
emetics for poisoning, 259
emphysema, pulmonary, 7, 10, 37
  subcutaneous, 2, 23, 30
emphysematous cystitis, 175
encephalitis, 10, 66, 112, 222, 241
endocardiosis, **49**
endocarditis, **49–40**, 241, 247
endocrine disorders, **203–24, 225–7**
  affecting the heart, 51, 55
  and diarrhoea, 135
  and polydipsia, **229**
  and weight loss, **233**
endoscope, 4, 103
  fibreoptic, 117, 141
endoscopy, 108, **117**
  see also Bronchoscopy; Proctoscopy
endotoxins, 54, 105, 126, 145, 159
enteritis, 105, **126**
  eosinophilic, 127, 135
  regional, 127, 135, 141
  and tenesmus, 189
enteropathy, protein-losing, 128, 193
eosinopenia, 213
eosinophilia, 11, 216
eosinophilic enteritis, 127
  pneumonia, 11

epilepsy, 65, 222, 258
  see also Convulsions; Seizures
epistaxis, 246
erythropoiesis, increased—see
  polycythaemia
  reduced, 165, **247**
escape beats, 70, 72
excitability, in poisoning, 257
exercise, excessive, 58, 234
  intolerance, 11, 45, 51, 59, 60, 61, 62,
    63, 207, 211, 213
  restriction, 7, 62, **93**, 152
  tolerance, 67
  unwillingness to, 17, 207
expectorants, 7
exploratory laparotomy, see Laparotomy
extrasystoles, see Tachydysrhythmias
exudative pericardidis, 52
pleurisy, **16**

'f' waves on ECG, 73
faecal coprophagy, 136
  culture, 137
  examination, 6, 132, **137**
    for Filaroides, 6, 43
  frequency, 136
  mucus, 136
  tenesmus, 177, 178, 179, **189–91**
  trypsin digest test, 137
faeces, blood (fresh), **133**, 136, 247
  consistency, 136
  minimal, 125
  undigested materials, 137
Fallot, see Tetralogy of Fallot
false pregnancy, see Pregnancy, false
Fanconi syndrome, 220, 230
fat assimilation test, 138
feminization, 217
fibreoptic endoscope, 38, 117, 141
fibrin degradation products, 246, 255
fibrinolytic agents in pleurisy, 20
Filaroides osleri (nodules), 1, 4, 5, 25, 26,
    27
  and airway obstruction, 1, 4
  larvae, 3, 6, 39
  radiology, 3
  treatment, 6
  fistula, recto-vaginal, 200
    ureterovaginal, 186, 200
flatulence, 136
fluid intake, normal, 229
fluid therapy,
  for acute abdominal disorders, 122

fluid therapy, (*cont.*)
  for acute intestinal disorders, 127
  for anaemia, 246, 252
  for cardiac failure, 63, 100
  causing cardiac decompensation, 58
  for diabetic ketoacidosis, 220
  for hypercalcaemia, 212
  for hypoadrenocorticalism, 217
  for pancreatitis, 160
  for poisonings, 260
  for pyometra, 228
  for renal failure, 164, 166
  in urinary obstruction, 173
fluoroscopy,
  abdominal, 201
  in airway obstruction, 3
  cardiac, 86
  gastric, 119
  oesophageal foreign body (for removal
    of), 103
  thoracic, 37
folate levels in malabsorption, 138
foreign body,
  abscess, 16, 241
  airway, 1, 3, 4, 16, 27, 30
  alimentary, 197
  anal, 189
  colonic, 131, 135, 137, 189, 199
  gastric, 105, 106, 107, 110, 118, 119,
    199
  intestinal, 113, 121, 125, 126, 131, 135,
    197
  oesophageal, 102, 103, 117, 118
  oral, 114
  penetrating, 241
  pharyngeal, 113, 114
  pleural, 16, 241
  rectal, 189
Fox terriers, 46
fracture (pelvic), 131
friction sounds, 32
fungal infections, *see* Mycosis

gallop rhythm, cardiac, 32, 59, 80
gammaglobulins,
  in autoimmune disease, 239
  in pyrexia, 243
gastric
  biopsy, 109, 119
  dilatation, 62, 105, 113, 119, 122,
    199
  disorders, acute, 105, 111
    chronic, 107, 111

gastric (*cont.*)
  and vomiting, 111, 113
  dysrhythmia, 105, 106
  enlargement, 193
  foreign body, 105, 107, 110,
    118, 119, 199
  infections, 105
  neoplasia, 107, 108, 118, 119, 198,
    246
  sedation, 106, 123
  stasis, 110
  torsion, 105
  ulceration, 105, 110, 118, 119, 199
  see also Pyloric disorders
gastritis, 105, 107, 113
  chronica, 107, 113
gastroenteritis, 121
  haemorrhagic, 105, 126, 258
gastrointestinal lavage, 260
  upsets, 121, 216
gastrotomy, 107, 108
genital disorders, 225–8
Giardia, 128, 129, 131, 135, 140
German shepherd dogs, 46, 51, 103, 117,
    136, 159, 203, 206, 234
globulin level, raised, 43, 147, 150, 239,
    243
glomerulonephritis, 17, 164, 165, 167
  in autoimmune disease, 167, 238, 239
  in weight loss, 234
glossitis, 114
glucagon, 160
  tolerance test, 222
glucocorticoid excess, 212, 218, 230
  insufficiency, 216
  therapy
    in acute abdominal disorders, 123
    for hypercalcaemia, 212
    in hypoadrenocorticalism, 217
    for hypoglycaemia, 222
  see also Corticosteroids
glucose absorption test, 138
  level, high, *see* Hyperglycaemia
    low, *see* Hypoglycaemia
  tolerance test, 219, 222
glycogen storage disease, 222
glycosides, cardiac,
  administration, 94–5
  for contractility, 92
  and gastric irritation, 105
  toxicity, 51, 95, 233
  withdrawal of, 73, 74
  see also Digitalization
glycosuria, 166, 218, 220, 230
goitre, 207, 209, 210

granulomatous diseases, 13, 16
  radiology, 36
  infections, 11, 13
  grass awns/seeds, 13, 16
Greyhounds, 12
growth hormone, excess, 206
  lack of, 203
growth, retarded—see stunted growth

haemangiosarcoma, 10, 12, 16, 51, 52
  146, 157, 192, 245
haemagglutination, 236, 237
haematemesis, 106, 107
haematology,
  in acute abdominal disorders, 122
  in anaemia, 250
  in cardiac failure, 89
  in diarrhoea, 138
  in haematuria, 184
  in haemolysis, 237, 248
  in haemorrhage, 253
  in hepatic disorders, 146
  in hyperadrenocorticalism, 213
  in hypothyroidism, 207
  in pulmonary disorders, 11
  in pyometra, 228
  in pyrexia, 243
  in respiratory disease, 43
  in thrombocytopenia, 238
haematuria, 171, 172, 174, 178, 179, 197,
  246
  differential diagnosis, 182
  investigation, 183
haemobartonellosis, 156, 248
haemoglobinura, 183, 236, 248
haemolytic anaemia, see Anaemia,
  haemolytic
haemopericardium, see Pericardial
  haemorrhage
haemoperitoneum, 192
haemophilia, 245
  diagnosis, 255
haemoptysis, 30
haemorrhage, acute, 245
  chronic, 246, 248
  intestinal, 126, 132, 133
  investigation of, 253
  petechial, 145, 253
  polydipsia and, 230
  prostatic, 179, 180
  pulmonary, 2, 22
  purpural, 213, 237
  thoracic, 16, 22

haemorrhage, (cont.)
  tracheal, 2
  treatment for, 246
  unaccountable, 252
  urinary, see Haematuria
haemorrhagic cystitis, 175
  diarrhoea (acute), 133
  gastroenteritis (HGE), 105, 110, 126,
  258
  shock, 145, 246
haemothorax, 16, 22
  therapy for, 20
heart 'attack', 63
  base tumour, 16, 18, 51, 52, 60
  beats, abnormal, see Dysrhythmias,
  cardiac
  blocks, 70, 72, 74
  rate, 32, 79
  slow, 72
  rhythm, see Rhythm, cardiac
  sounds, see Sounds, cardiac
  see also Cardiac disorders
heart–lung machine, 92
heat stroke, 10, 27, 258
hepatic amyloidosis, 147
  biopsy, 146, 148, 150, 151
  cirrhosis, 146, 150, 192
  disorders, 144–54
  diagnosis, 149
  management, 152
  encephalopathy, 144, 147, 151, 152
  enlargement, 52, 53, 60, 84, 148, 153,
  193, 213, 218, 236
  failure, acute, 145
  chronic, 113, 146, 233
  and haemorrhage, 144, 147, 151, 245
  polydipsia, 230
  insufficiency and maldigestion, 135
  neoplasia, 113, 146, 149, 150, 153,
  192, 242
  radiology, 147, 148, 151, 196, 197, 201
  trauma, 145
  see also Jaundice
hepatitis, chronic, active, 146
  toxic, 145
  vasculitis and, 246
  viral, 105, 113, 122, 145, 149, 246, 258
hepatomegaly, see Hepatic enlargement
  differential diagnosis, 158
hernia, diaphragmatic, see Diaphragm,
  ruptured
  pericardiodiaphragmatic, 18, 46, 92
  perineal, 7, 131, 172, 189
  strangulated, 122, 125
  ventral, 194

herpes virus, 5
hiatus hernia, 102, 103, 114, 119
Hickey Hare test, 232
hookworms, 128, 247
hormonal disorders, *see* Endocrine
    disorders
Horner's syndrome, 30
HPOA, 11, 19, 31
hydralazine, 91, **94**, 97
hydronephrosis, 163, 165, 173
hydrothorax, **16–18**, 26, 35, **40**, 60
    treatment, **40**
hyperadrenocorticalism, 149, 153, 194,
    212, 218, 229, 235
    iatrogenic, 212
    treatment, 214
hyperaesthesia, 210, 258
hyperammonaemia, 66, 151
hypercalcaemia, 163, **212**, 216
hypercalcitonism, **210**
hyperglycaemia, 147, 151, 206, 213, 218,
    219
hyperkalaemia, 53, 65, 72, 166, 173
hyperlipidosis, 149, 160
hyperparathyroidism, 165, **211**
hyperpnoea, 25
hypersexuality, 217
hyperthermia, 27
hyperthyroidism, 27, 55, **209**, 242
    iatrogenic, 209
hypertrophic osteoarthropathy, *see* HPOA
hypoadrenocorticalism, 37, 53, 54, 85,
    113, 122, 212, **215**, 219, 222, 258
    and anaemia, 247
hypoalbuminaemia, 43, 147, 150, 168
hypocalcaemia, **54**, **66**, 166, 210, **211**,
    222, 258
    in dysrhythmias, 72
hypoglycaemia, 65, 147, 151, 216, 220,
    221
    differential diagnosis, **222**
hypokalaemia, **54**, 66
hyponatraemia, 66, 216
hypoparathyroidism, 54, **210**
hypophysectomy, 215
hypopituitarism, **203**
hypoproteinaemia, 10, 17, 43, 52, 64, 66,
    89, 144, 147, 150, 168, 193, 235,
    246
hypotension, 93, 99
hypotensive drugs, *see* Vasodilator
    therapy
hypothermia,
    in acute abdominal disorders, 121
    in dyspnoea, 31

hypothermia, (*cont.*)
    in dysrhythmias, 72
    in endocrine disorders, 207, 215
    effect on heart, 99
    in poisoning, 257, 258
    in renal failure, 164
hypothyroidism, 55, 149, **206**, 215, 235
    and anaemia, 247
    diagnosis, 207
    treatment, 208
hypovascular lungs, 36, 85
hypovalaemia, 37, 54, 62, 85, 99, 163,
    216, 246
    effect of diuresis, 93
    see also Shock, hypovolaemic
hypoxia, cerebral, 63
    in dysrhythmias, 72
    effect on heart, 99
    myocardial, 54
    see also Cyanosis

iatrogenic
    acromegaly, 206, 230
    diabetes mellitus, 218
    gastritis, 105
    hyperadrenocorticalism, 212, 230
    hyperthyroidism, 209, 230
    hypoadrenocorticalism, 216
    hypoglycaemia, 220
    marrow depression, 245, **247**, 249
    polydipsia, 230
    poisoning, 113, 258
    weight loss, 233
    see also corticosteroids, glycosides,
        insulin, oestrogens, phenothiazines,
        phenylbutazone, phenytoin,
        primidone, progestogens,
        salicylates, vasodilators
icterus, *see* Jaundice
ileus (paralytic), 113, 122, 126, 129, 159
immunization, *see* Vaccination
immunosuppressive drugs, 168, **237**, 243
inappetance, 6, 11, 12, 30, 50, 102, 106,
    107, 119, 121, 125, 128, 145, 147,
    160, 161, 164, 165, 178, 211. 216,
    225, 228, 233, 236, 242
incontinence, urinary, 170, 171, 179
    differential diagnosis, **185**
    hormonal, 185, 187, 226
    investigation, **186**
    paradoxical, 185
    treatment, **187**
incoordination, 221, 258

infarction, myocardial, 51
  and pyrexia, 242
infections, causing pyrexia, **241**
  see also under individual organs
infectious canine hepatitis, see Hepatitis,
  viral
inhalation, of fumes, 10
  pneumonia, 10, 103, 120
inotropic drugs, 52, 63, 97
insulin, administration, **220-21**
  antagonists, 218, 222
  excess, 54, **221**
  level, high, 221
  stabilization, 221
insulinoma, see Islet cell tumour
interstitial nephritis, 163, 165
  pneumonia, 12
intervertebral disc, prolapsed, 66, 186
intestinal absorbants, **141**, 260
  bacterial overgrowth, 127
  biopsy, 140
  'carrier' failures, 127, 135
  chronic disorders, **127-9**
  foreign body, 113, 121, 125, 127, 131,
    135, 197
  linear, 127, 199
  haemorrhage, 126, 128, 132, **133**
  infections, 126, 131
  treatment, 132
  irritation, **126**
  malabsorption, 134, **135**, 138, 141, 193,
    210
  maldigestion, 127, 134
  motility, 134
  neoplasia, 113, 122, 125, 127, 129,
    131, 135, 149, 233, 246
  obstruction, 111, 113, 121, **125**
  radiology, **197**, 198, 199
  parasites, 119, 123, **128**, 131, 135
  treatment, **128**
  rupture, **126**, 192, 241
  sedatives, 127, **141**
  torsion, 113, 125
intestine, large, disorders, **131-3**, 136, **141**
  small, disorders, **125-9**, 136, **137**
intravenous
  fluids, see Fluid therapy
  urography, 174, **184**, 187, 191, **200**
intussusception, 113, 121, **125**, 126, 127,
    133, 136, 189, 199
Irish setters, 29, 102, 117, 127, 206,
    234
iron deficiency and anaemia, 247, 248
  therapy, 249, 251
'irritable colon', 130, 132, 133

islet cell tumour, **221**
isoprenaline, **74**, 100

jaundice, 145, 147, 150, 161, 236, 248
  differential diagnosis, **155-6**
  investigation of, **156**
joint pain, 50, 211, 238, 242

Keeshond, 46
kennel cough, 5, 27
  treatment, 6, 7
ketoacidosis, 218, 220
kidneys, mis-shapen, 166
  see also Renal disorders

laboratory tests,
  in abdominal enlargement, 195
  in acute abdominal disorders, **122-3**
  in anaemia, **249-50**, 251, **254-5**
  in autoimmune disorders, 237, 238, 239
  in cardiac failure, 89
  in chronic diarrhoea, **137-40**
  for collapse, **67**
  in endocrine disorders, 204, 205, 207,
    210, 212, 213-5, 216, 219, 222
  in haematuria, **184**
  in hepatic disorders, 145, 147, **149-51**
  in jaundice, **156**
  in pancreatitis, **160**
  in pleural effusions, 18, **40-42**
  in polydipsia, **231-2**
  in pyometra, 228
  in pyrexia, **243**
  in renal failure, 164, **166**, 168
  in respiratory disease, 43
  in urinary disorders, 171, 173, 175
  in vomiting, 117
  in weight loss, **234-5**
  see also Bacteriology; Biopsy;
    Cytology; Haematology; Urinalysis
lactase insufficiency, 135
lactation, 225, 230
  tetany, see Eclampsia
lactulose in hepatic encephalopathy, 152
lameness, 19, 50, 242
laparotomy, exploratory,
  in abdominal enlargement, 195
  in abdominal haemorrhage, 246
  in gastric lesions, 108, 119

laparotomy, (*cont.*)
  in haematuria, 184
  in hepatic disorders, 149, 151
  in pancreatitis, 160
  in prostatic disorders, 180
  in tenesmus, 191
laryngeal,
  collapse, 1
  disorders, 1
  diagnosis, 3
  neoplasia, 1
  paralysis, 1, 4
laryngitis, 5
laryngoscopy, 3, 39
lavage, gastrointestinal, in poisoning,
    259
laxatives, 133
LE cell preparation, 239
leishmaniasis, 155, 248
leptospirosis, 105, 145, 155, 163, 165,
    182, 248
leucocytosis, in bronchopneumonia, 11
  in endocarditis, 50
  in pyometra, 228
  in pyrexia, 243
leukaemias, 157, 204, 247, 250
  and pyrexia, 242
  and weight loss, 233
lignocaine, 73, **75**, 100
lipaemia, 219
lipase level, in pancreatitis, 160
liver,
  enzyme levels, 89, 123, 145, 147,
    149–150, 206, 213, 219
  fatty degeneration/infiltration, **148**,
    213
  function tests, 150
  size,
    large—*see* hepatic enlargement
    small, 147
  see also Hepatic disorders
lung, *see* Pulmonary
lupus erythematosus, systemic, **238**,
    242
lymphangiectasia, 17, 127, 135
lymphatics, obstruction, 16, 64
  traumatic rupture, 16, 193
lymph node biopsy, 243
lymphomegaly,
  abdominal—on radiographs, 196
  and airway obstruction, 1
  in autoimmune disease, 236, 237, 238,
    250
  in respiratory disease, 18, 30
lymphopenia, 166, 213

lymphosarcoma, and anaemia, 247
  cardiac, 51
  hepatic, 146
  and hypercalcaemia, 211
  intestinal, 127, 135, 140
  pulmonary, 12
  and pyrexia, 242
  splenic, 157
  thymic, 2, 18
  and weight loss, 233

malabsorption, 17, 134, **135**, 138, 139,
    140, 193, 210
  and anaemia, 138, 248
  tests, 125–7, **137–40**
  treatment for, 141
  in weight loss, 233
maldigestion, 127, 134
  and anaemia, 248
  in weight loss, 233
mammary enlargement, 225
  neoplasia, 12, 233
mandible fracture, 114
  luxation, 114
Marie's disease, *see* HPOA
marrow, bone, biopsy, 243, 251
  depression, 245, **247**
  exhaustion, 248
  nutritional deficiency, **248**
mediastinal abscesses, 18
  disorders, **16–19**
  effusions, 16, 17
  neoplasms, 18, 42, 114
  radiography, 34, **35**
mediastinitis, 16
  see also Pneumomediastinum
megacolon, 131, 132, 189
megaloesophagus, *see* Oesophageal
    dilatation
malaena, 107, 246
melanosis—*see* skin pigmentation
meningitis and collapse, 66
metabolic disorders,
  affecting CNS, **65**
  the heart, 51, **53**
  endocrine 203–24
  and weight loss, 233
metastases, *see* Neoplasia
methaemoglobinaemia, 68
metoclopramide, 103, 115, 123
metoestrus, 206, 218, 225, 227
metronidazole, 19, 129
microbiology, *see* Bacteriology

microcardia, 54, 216
milk intolerance, see Disaccharidase insufficiency
mineralocorticoid insufficiency, see Hypoadrenocorticalism
misalliance, 227
misdosing, 2
'missed' beats, 72
mitral valve dysplasia, 46, 48
  endocardiosis, 49
  incompetence, 49, 58, 63
mucolysis, in airway disorders, 7
mucous membranes, blue—see cyanosis
  pale, 11, 17, 23, 62, 99, 207, 236, 246, 250
  ulcerated, 165
murmurs, cardiac, 32, 47, 59, 60, 63
  character, 80–82
  congenital, 47
  diastolic, 50, 82
  false, 80
  haemic, 80, 243, 250
  intensity, 80
  'machinery', 48, 82
  and phonocardiography, 82
  sites, 47, 80
  systolic, 46, 47, 82
muscle enzymes, 89
  relaxants, 39, 103
  tremor, 210, 221, 225, 258
  see also neuromuscular disorders
myasthenia gravis, 18, 66, 102, 114, 239
mycosis, 11, 13, 241
myeloma, 211, 242, 247
myocardial activity, assessment, 89
  contractility, assessment, 89, 90
    increased, 57
    reduced, 51, 54, 62, 63, 75
    therapy, 52, 92, 95, 96
  contusion, 22, 51
  dilatation, 50
  disease, 50, 54, 60, 63, 71, 72, 74, 75
    effect on rhythm, 71–3
    and muscle enzymes, 89
  failure, 51, 58, 61
  fibrosis, 50
  hypertrophy, 52, 57, 75
  hypoxia, 51, 57, 62
  infarction, 50, 51, 63
  irritability, 75
  ischaemia, 50, 62
  neoplasia, 51
  rupture, 50
  toxins, 54, 62

myocardial, (cont.)
  trauma, 23, 50
  see also Cardiomyopathy
myocarditis, 50, 241
myopathies, 65, 66
myositis, temporal, 114

narcolepsy, 65
nares, stenotic, 1
nasal discharge, 6, 11, 112
neoplasia, 246
nebulization for airway disorders, 7
neoplasia,
  abdominal, 111, 192, 193, 194, 217, 227, 233
  adrenal, 212, 215, 216, 217
  airway, 1, 3, 26
  and anaemia, 245, 246, 247
  bile duct, 146, 149
  bladder, 172, 174, 182, 190, 246
  carcinoma, 12, 146, 211, 222, 233, 242
  carcinomatosis, 17, 193, 227, 233
  cardiac, 51, 62
  colonic, 131, 133, 137, 189, 199
  and effusions, 16–18, 41–2
  gastric, 107, 108, 119, 198, 246
  'heart base', 16, 18, 51, 52, 60
  hepatic, 113, 146, 148, 149, 153, 194, 222, 242
  intestinal, 113, 122, 125, 127, 129, 131, 149, 233, 246
  laryngeal, 1
  mammary, 12, 233
  mediastinal, 18, 42, 114
  melanomas, 12
  mesothelioma, 17, 193
  metastatic, 11, 12, 14, 33, 51, 146, 212
    radiology, 36
  myeloma, 211, 247
  myocardial, 51
  nasal, 246
  and obstruction of lymphatics, 16
    venous return, 16, 31, 62, 64, 148, 193
  oesophageal, 102, 114, 118
  oral, 114
  osteosarcomas, 12
  ovarian, 193, 194, 227
  pancreatic, 113, 149, 159, 161, 221
  parathyroid, 211
  penis, 172, 174, 183
  pituitary, 205, 206, 212

neoplasia, (*cont.*)
  pleural, 16–18
  prostatic, 172, 174, **178**, 182, 190,
    200
  and pyrexia, **242**
  and weight loss, **233**
  pulmonary, **10**, 12, 13, 26, 28, 35, 36,
    39, 42, 233
  renal, 163, 165, 182, 197, 200
  splenic, **157**
  testicular, 179, 194, 215
  thoracic, 2
  thymic, 2, 18
  thyroid, 1, 207, **209**
  tonsillar, 1, 114
  vaginal, 172, 174, 183, 186, 190, 200
  see also Haemangiosarcoma;
    Leukaemias; Lymphosarcoma
nephritis, *see* Renal failure
nephrogenic diabetes insipidus, **205**, 231
nephrotic syndrome, 17, 64, **167**, 193,
  234
  see also Renal failure
nerve dysfunction, and collapse, **66**
nervousness, *see* Psychological disorders
neuromuscular disorders, and weakness,
  66, 93, 207, 213
neutropenia, 239, 241, 247
Newfoundlands, 46
nocardiosis, 16, 192, 241
  therapy for, 19
noise, respiratory, *see* Respiratory noise
normoblasts in anaemia, 250

obesity, 153, 159, 194, 207
  and cardiac disease, 55, 58, 91
  differential diagnosis, **235**
oculonasal discharge, 6
oedema, of head, 31, 209
  pulmonary, *see* Pulmonary oedema
  subcutaneous, 18, 31, 60, **64**, 128,
    167
oesophageal dilatation, 2, 10, 18, 102,
  117, 118, 119
  disorders, **102**, 113, 114
  management, **103**
  diverticulum, 102, 118, 119
  fistula, 103
  foreign body, 102, **103**, 117, 118, 119
  neoplasia, 102, 114, 118
  obstruction, 2
  perforation, 16, 17, 103, 118
  radiology, **118**

oesophageal dilation, (*cont.*)
  stricture, 102, 103, 118, 119
  ulceration, 103
oesophagitis, 102, 113, 114, 117, 118
  treatment, 103
oesophagotomy, 103
oesophagus, flaccid, 103
  fluid, 117
oestrogens, excess, 178, 179, **226**, 227,
  245, 247
  for false pregnancy, 226
  for incontinence, **187**
  lack of, in spayed bitches, 185, 187,
    226
  for prostatic disease, 177–**80**
oestrus, abnormal, 183, 217, 226, 227
  in polydipsia, 230
  prolonged, 227
  see also Anoestrus
oligaemia, *see* Anaemia
oliguria, 123, **164**, 175
opiates, 8, 24, 97, 112, 122, 123, 133,
  141, 160
oral foreign body, 114
  neoplasia, 114
  ulceration, 12, 258
orthopaedic,
  disorders, causing weakness, 66
  resulting from hypercalcitonism, 210
orthopnoea, 25, 30
osmolality, plasma, **232**
  urine, 205, **232**
ossification, epiphyseal, delayed, 204
osteodystrophy, fibrous, 114, 165
  hypertrophic, 241
osteomyelitis,
  in hypercalcaemia, 212
  in pyrexia, 241
osteopathy, craniomandibular, 114
osteoporosis, 114, 211, **212**, 213
osteosarcoma, 12
otitis media, and weakness, 66
ovarian cyst, 193, 226, **227**
  disorders, **225–7**
  imbalance, 215, 217, **226**
  neoplasia, 193, 194, **227**
ovariohysterectomy, 206, 220, 226, 227,
  228
  effect on incontinence, 185, 226
oxygen therapy, 3
  in cardiac arrest, 100
  in cardiac failure, 92
  in pulmonary disorders, 13
  in thoracic trauma, 23
  venous level, 60, 68

P wave (in ECG), absent, 72, 73
  dissociated from QRS, 72
  premature, 73
  suppressed, 54, 73, 216
  waveform change, 73
PABA test, 140
pacemaker, artificial, **74**
  depression, 72
  dominant, 70
  ectopic, 70
  substitute, 70
pain, *see* Abdominal pain; Joint pain
  in pyrexia, 242
pallor, *see* Mucous membranes, pale
palpation, abdominal, 117, 122, 126, 132,
    137, 171, 172, 174, 180, 183,
    190, 194
  of neck, 117
  of pharynx, 117
  rectal, *see* Rectal examination
pancreatic degenerative atrophy, 159
  disorders, **159–61**
  endocrine disorders, **217–22**
  exocrine insufficiency, 135, 138, 140,
    159, 161, 218
  tests, **137–40**
  therapy, **142**
  extract, 142, 152
  hypoplasia, 159
  neoplasia, 113, 149, 159, **161, 221**
pancreatitis, 66, 113, 122, 149, **159**, 192,
    211
  therapy for, medical, **160**
  surgical, 123, 160
papain test, 237
paracentesis, *see* Abdominal paracentesis;
    Pericardiocentesis; Thoracentesis
parainfluenza, 5
paralysis, spinal, and weakness, 66
  and constipation, 131
paraprostatic cyst, 179
paraquat poisoning, 10, **12**, 14, 27, 102,
    163, **258**
parasitic infections, and anaemia, 247
  intestinal, **128**, 131, 135
  respiratory, 12, 13
  treatment, 6, **14, 128**
  and weight loss, 204, 234
parathyroid disorders, **190**, 210
paroxysmal tachycardias, 73, 75
parturition,
  and dyspnoea, 27
  false, 225
  and genital tenesmus, 190
parvovirus, 59, 105, 113, 126, 258

patent ductus arteriosus, 45, 46, 48
  surgery, 92
Pekingeses, 49
pelvic fracture, 131, 189
pemphigus vulgaris, 239
penile neoplasia, 172, 174, 183
  trauma, 172, 183
peptic ulcer, 105, 107, 108, 118, 119, 192,
    199
percussion, thoracic, 17, 18, 23, **31**, 79
perianal fistulae, 189
periarteritis—*see* polyarteritis
pericardial disease, **52**
  congenital, 46, 47
  effusion, **52**, 58, 60, 91
    treatment, **92**
  haemorrhage, 22, 52, 58
  trauma, 52
pericardiocentesis, 61, **92**
pericardiodiaphragmatic hernia, 18, **46**
  surgery, 92
pericarditis, 52, 241
perineal hernia, 7, 131, 172, 173, 189,
    190
periosteal haemorrhage, 241
peritoneal dialysis, 164
  disorders, **192–5**
  effusions, **192–5**
  haemorrhage, **192**
peritonitis, 113, 122, 126, 129, 145, 159,
    178, **192**, 241
peritracheal masses, 1
petechial haemorrhages, 145, 253
phaeochromocytoma, 27, **217**, 218, 219,
    242
pharyngeal examination, 2
  foreign body, 113, 114
  inco-ordination, 102, 113
  palpation, 117
  retching, **112**, 113
pharyngitis, 5, 113, 114
phenothiazines, 145, 152, 244, 245
phenylbutazone, 237, 245, 247
phenytoin, 152, 245, 247
phonocardiography, 82, **87**
phosphorus level, abnormal, 166, **212**
physiotherapy for pulmonary disorders,
    7
pigmentation, of skin, 204, 207, 213
pituitary disorders, **203**
  dwarfism, 203
  neoplasia, 205, 206, 212
plasma levels, *see* under individual
    constituents
  volume, increase, 57

platelet counts, 254
  disorders, 16, 184, **245**
  function tests, 238, 254
  see also Thrombocytopenia
pleural disorders, **16–21**
  effusion, **16–18**, 167
  therapy, **19–20**
  foreign body, 16, 241
  radiology, **35**
  tumours, 16–19
pleurisy, 16, 241, 247
pneumocolography, 132, 141, 191, **199**
pneumocystogram, 171, 173, 174, 175,
    184, 191, **199**
pneumomediastinum, 17
pneumonia, allergic (eosinophilic), 11,
    27
  treatment, 14
  inhalation, 10, 27, 103, 120
  interstitial, 12, 258
  radiology, **36**
  viral, 12
  see also Bronchopneumonia;
    Pulmonary disorders
pneumoperitoneum, 193
pneumothorax, 17, 22, 40
  radiology, **35**
  therapy, 20, 40
poisoning, acute, **257–61**
  alphachloralose, 257
  antidotes, **260**
  chlorinated hydrocarbons, 258
  common, **257**
  glycol, 66, 145, 163, 258, 260
  heavy metal, 66, 122, 145, 163
  lead, 105, 222, 247, 258, 260
  management, **260**
  metaldehyde, 258
  organophosphates, 105, 258
  paraquat, 10, 12, 14, 102, 163, 258, 260
  sodium chlorate, 260
  strychnine, 258, 260
  warfarin, 16, **245**, 255, 257, 260
poisons, alimentary, 113, 122
  detoxification, by liver, 144
  in hepatic failure, 145
polyarteritis nodosa, 239, 242, 246
polyarthritis, autoimmune, 238, 239
polycythaemia, 11, 68, 89
polydipsia, 147, 165, 205, 206, 209, 211,
    213, 216, 218, 228, **229**
  differential diagnosis, **229–32**
  endocrine, 229
  iatrogenic, 230
  investigation, **230–32**

polydipsia, (cont.)
  psychogenic, 230
  and weight loss, 234
polyphagia, 209, 213, 218, 225
polyuria, 165, 186, 205, 209, 211, 213,
    218, 228, **229–32**
Pomeranians, 46
Poodles, miniature, 46, 49, 213, 218
portal venography, **201**
portosystemic shunts, 146, 151, 201
potassium level, depressed, see
    Hypokalaemia
  elevated, see Hyperkalaemia
  in hypoadrenocorticalism, 216
  supplementation, in diuresis, 93
P–Q interval, prolonged, 211, 216
Prazosin, 91, **94**
precordial thrill, 48, 79
pregnancy,
  and abdominal enlargement, 193
  in cardiac disease, 58, 62
  diagnosis, 197
  and dyspnoea, 26
  false, 27, 225, 226, 227
  prevention, 91
  and weight loss, 234
premature beats, see Beats, premature
primidone, 145, 151, 152,
proctoscopy, 132, **141**, 191
progestogens, excess, **206**, 218, 226, 230
  for false pregnancy, 226
  in pyometra, 227
prolapse, rectal, 132
pro-oestrus, prolonged, 183, 227
propranolol–see β-adrenergic blockade
prostaglandin therapy, 226, 228
prostatectomy, 178
prostatic abscessation, 177, **178**, 181
  biopsy, 180
  cysts, **179**, 200
  disorders, 172, **177–81**, 182, 186, 189
  enlargement, **177–9**, 184, 189, 190
  haemorrhage, 177, 179, 182
  neoplasia, 172, 174, **178**, 182, 190, 200
  pain, 171, 178
  treatment, 178, **180**
prostatitis, 122, 170, 172, **177**, 241
protein intake,
  in hepatic failure, 152
  in renal failure, 166, 168
protein level, low, see Hypoproteinaemia
protein-losing effusions, 43
  enteropathy, 17, 64, **127**, 193, 234
  nephropathy, 17, 64, **167**, 193, 234
proteinuria, 166, **168**

prothrombin time, **255**
pseudocyesis, **225**
pseudohyperparathyroidism, **211**, 212
psychogenic diarrhoea, 136
  dyspnoea, 27
  incontinence, 186
  polydipsia, 230, 231
  syncope, 66
  vomiting, 112, 113, 115, 119
  weight loss, 234
psychological disturbances, 225
pulmonary
  abscess, 13, 35, 36
  alveolar disorders, **10**
  biopsy, 12, **42**
  bullae, 12, 13, 17, 37
  collapse, 10, 13, 35
  emphysema, 7, **11**, 26, 37
  exudation, **10**
  haemorrhage, 2, **10**, 20, 26
  hypertension, 45, 53
  hypervascularity, 37
  hypovascularity, 36, **85**
  infections, 10, 11, 12, 13, 14
  interstitial disease, **12**, 53
  neoplasia, **10, 12**, 13, 26, 28, 33, 35,
    36, 42, 233
  oedema, 2, **10**, 12, 26, 27, **58, 84**
    treatment, 4, 14, **93**, 96
  radiography, 11, 12, **35–6**, 84
  radiology, 35–6
  rupture, 12
  sounds, *see* Sounds, respiratory
  torsion, 12, 13, 16
  trauma, 10, 14, **22**
  vascular disorders, 13, 16, 53
pulmonic stenosis, **46**, 60, 63, 88
  surgery for, 92
pulse,
  absence, 62, 78, 99
  character, **78**
  deficit, 72, 73, 78
  in dysrhythmias, 51, 71, 72, 73
  hard, 165
  pressure, 79
  quality, **77**
  rate, 51, 61, 73, **78**
  strong, 50, 72, 78
  variable, 73, 78, 160
  weak, 51, 59, 61, 62, 73, 78, 216, 236,
    250
PUO, *see* Pyrexia
puppies, anaemia, 248
  see also Congenital disorders
Purkinje system, 70

purpura, 237, 253
pyelogram,
  intravenous—*see* urography
pyelonephritis, 163, 165, 170, 182, 241
pyloric dysfunction, 105, **107**, 108, 113,
  199
  function assessment, 119
  obstruction, 105, 106, 113
  stenosis, 105, **107**, 113, 119, 199
pyloromyotomy, 108
pyoderma, 207, 218
pyometra, 51, 113, 183, 192, 193, 197,
  227, 229, 241, 247
  diagnosis, 197, **228**
  treatment, 228
pyothorax, **16, 19**, 241, 247
  see also Pleurisy
pyrexia, 31, 50, 103, 121, 126, 145,
  164, 178, 210, 228, 230, 238
  differential diagnosis, **241–2**
  investigation of, **242–4**
  see also Antipyretics
pyruvate kinase deficiency, 248
pyuria, 50, 178, 180, 243

QRS complex (ECG) absence, 72
  dissociated from P wave, 72, 73
  irregular, 73
  premature, 73
  variations, 72, 73
Q–T interval short, 211
quinidine sulphate, 73, **75**

rabies, 114
radiography,
  abdominal, **196–7**
  alimentary, upper, **118**
  contrast media, *see* Angiography;
    Barium; Bronchography;
    Cystography; Pneumocolography;
    Pneumocystogram; Urography
  hepatic, 148, 151
  thoracic, **33–4**
  see also Fluoroscopy; Tomography
radioisotopes, in cardiac investigation, 90
  in hypothyroidism, 208
radiology,
  abdominal, 122, 194, **196–202**
  airway, 3, 34, **36**,
  alimentary, **118, 197, 198, 199**
  bladder, 171, 173, 174, 175, 196, 197,
    199, 200

radiology, (*cont.*)
  cardiac, 60, 61, 62, **83–6**
  colonic, 141, 196, **199**
  in congenital cardiac disease, 48
  for effusions, 35, 197
  in false pregnancy, 225
  gastric, 108, 118, **198**
  hepatic, 147, 148, 151, 196, 197, **201**
  in hyperadrenocorticalism, 213
  in incontinence, 187
  mediastinal, 19, **35**
  oesophageal, 19, 34, **118**
  pericardial, 52
  pleural, 18, 19, **35**
  prostatic, 179, **180**, 196, 199, **200**
  pulmonary, **35–6**
  in pyometra, 228
  in pyrexia, 243
  renal, 163, **198**
  in tenesmus, **191**, 197
  thoracic, 10, 16, **33–7**, 50
  urinary, 171, 173, 174, 175, 184, 187, 197, **199–200**
  in vomiting, 118, 122
râles, respiratory, 11, **32**, 59, 82
RBC in anaemia, 248, **250**
  fragility, 248
rectal examination,
  in colonic disorders, 132
  in diarrhoea, 137
  in haematuria, 184
  in prostatic disease, **180**
  in tenesmus, **190**
  in urinary disease, 171, 173, 174
rectal foreign body, 137, 189
  prolapse, 132
  sacculation, 189, 199
  stricture, 189
rectal—*see also* colonic
reflux, duodenal-gastric, 110
regurgitation, 5, 10, 18, 102, **112**
  differential diagnosis, **113**
  in thyroid neoplasia, 209
  in weight loss, 233
renal amyloidosis, 165, 167
  biopsy, 164, 166, 168, 239
  calculi, 163
  clearance tests, 166
  disorders, **163–9**, 182
  dysplasia, 165, 199, 200
  failure, acute, **163**, 182, 258
    and cardiac disease, 54, 58
    chronic, 51, 113, **165**, 210, 229, 233, 247
    compensated, 165, 229
    decompensating, 165, 229

renal failure, (*cont.*)
  and gastric disorders, 107
  laboratory findings, 164, 166, 168
  and poisoning, 163, 258
  treatment, 164, 166, 168
  neoplasia, 163, 165, 182, 197, 200
  perfusion, decreased, 57, 163
  radiology, 163, **200**
  trauma, 163, 182
respiration, artificial, 3
  character, 25
respiratory arrest, 99
  depression, 24
  disorders, effect on heart, 58, 70
  differential diagnosis, **25–28**
  investigation, **29–44**
  emergency, 3
  infections, **5**
  noise, 2, 18, 22, **26**, **28**, 59, 206
  rate (normal), 31
  sounds, 6, 11, **32**
    displaced, 17, 23
    muffled, 23
  see also Airway disorders; Pulmonary disorders
resuscitation, **99–101**
retching, 110, **112**
  differential diagnosis, **113**
reticulocytes, in anaemia, 250
Retrievers, 206
rheumatoid arthritis, 239, 242
rhinitis, 5, 6
rhonchi, 6, 11, **32**, 82
rhythm, cardiac, 'chaotic', **70**
  normal, 73
  gallop, 32, 59, **80**
  see also Dysrhythmias, cardiac
ribs, fractured, 22
'roarer' *see* Laryngeal paralysis
'rubber jaw' 114, 165
ruptured diaphragm, 17, 18, **22**, 26, 30, 35

salicylate,
  therapy, 141, 237, 243
  toxicity, 105, 108, 112, 245
salivary cyst, 1
salivation, 110, 112
  excess, 102, 258
salmonellae, 126, 131, 132, 135, 145
salt-free diet, **94**, 152, 168
salt supplementation, in diet, 171, 173, 217, 230
Samoyeds, 218

samples, blood, *see* Blood sampling;
    Haematology
urine, *see* Urinalysis
scavenging, 119, 134, 137, 258
Scottish type terriers, 102, 107, 117
seborrhoea, 207, 218, 226
sedation, in cardiac failure, 96, 97
    in false pregnancy, 226
    gastric, 106, 123
    in poisoning, 261
seizure, 147, 210, 221, **222**, 258
    differential diagnosis, **222**
sepsis,
    and anaemia, 247
    and embolism, 51
    and the heart, 50, 51, 58
    internal, 241
    and poor growth, 204
    and pyrexia, **241**, 243
    and shock, 62, 66
    and weight loss, 233
septal defects, cardiac, 46
Sertoli cell tumour, 178, 179
sexual behaviour, and adrenal gland, 217
SGOT, *see* AST
SGPT, *see* ALT
Shigella, 126, 135
shock, 23, 27, 37, 54, 106, 121, 126,
    145, 159
    cardiogenic, 51, **61–3**
    electric, 10
    endotoxic, 105, 126, 159
    effect on the heart, 58, 62, 99
    hypovolaemic, 163, 216, 246
        treatment, 122, 164, 217, 246
    neurogenic, 62
    septic, 62
shunts, arteriovenous, 64
    pulmonary, 13
    cardiovascular, 63
    left-to-right, 36, **45**, 61
    portosystemic, 146, 151, 201
    right-to-left, 36, **45**, 63, 85
sino-atrial block, 72
sinus
    arrest, 70, **71**, 74
    arrhythmia, **70**, 71, 72, 74
    bradycardia, 72, 74
    rhythm, 70, 78
    tachycardia, **70**
skeletal density (loss of)—*see*
    osteoporosis
skin, lesions, in lupus erythematosus,
    238
    pigmentation, 207, 213

SLE, *see* Lupus erythematosus, systemic
smoke inhalation, 5, 10, 25
sneeze, reverse, 6
sodium, dietary restriction, 94, 168
    levels, in hypoadrenocorticalism, 216
    see also hyponatraemia
soft palate, elongated, 1
    surgery, 4
sounds, adventitious, **32**
    alimentary, 23, 126, 136
    cardiac, **79–82**
        area increased, 59, **79**
        audibility, 32, 79
        displaced, 19, 23, 79
        inaudible, 32, 99
        muffed, 11, 17, 19, 23, 32, 52, 62, **79**
        and phonocardiography, 87
        in respiratory disease, 32
        in tachydysrhythmias, 72–3
    crepitant, 32
    friction, 32, 80
    respiratory, 6, 11, **32**
    vesicular, 11, 32
    see also Murmurs; Râles; Rhonchi
spasmolytic drugs, 123
spayed bitches, hormone imbalance, 185,
    226
spaying—*see* ovariohysterectomy
Spirocerca lupi, 102
splenectomy, 158, 237, 248
splenic disorders, **157**
    hyperplasia, 157
    neoplasia, 113, **157**, 193
    torsion, 122, 157, 193, 242
splenomegaly, 60, **157**, 193, 250
    in autoimmune disease, 236, 237, 238
spinal disorders, in incontinence, 186
    in weakness, 66
    see also CNS disorders
stagnant bowel loop, 134, 136
stiffness, 238, 242
stomach tube, in dilatation, 106
    see also Gastric disorders
stomatitis, 114
storage diseases, 65, 147, 222
stroke volume, increased, 57
stunted growth,
    in congenital cardiovascular disorders,
        45, 47
    differential diagnosis, **204**
    in hypothyroidism, 206
    in panhypopituitarism, 203
    in portosystemic shunts, 148
subaortic stenosis, *see* Aortic stenosis
sudden death, 99, 216, 261

surgery,
for airway obstruction, 4
blood transfusions, **252**
for congenital cardiac defects, **92**
in diabetes mellitus, 221
for *Filaroides osleri*, 6
for gastric disorders, 107, 109
for hyperadrenocorticalism, 215
for hyperparathyroidism, 212
for incontinence, 187, 188
for islet cell tumour, 222
mediastinal, 19
for oesophageal lesions, 103
for pancreatitis, 123, 160
pleural, 19
prostatic, 178
pulmonary, 13
for ruptured diaphragm, 20, 23
for thoracic trauma, 23
for thoracic duct, 20
for tracheal collapse, 4
and urinary obstruction, 173, 175
for vaginal neoplasms, 174
for vascular ring strictures, 92
see also—castration, laparotomy
    exploratory, ovariohysterectomy,
    splenectomy, thoracotomy,
    tracheotomy
surgical haemorrhage, 245
infection, 16, 241
swallow, attempts, 112
barium, 37, **118**
(discomfort on swallowing), 112
failure, 102
syncope, *see* Collapse
systemic lupus erythematosus, **238**
systolic murmurs, *see* Murmurs, systolic
time intervals, 90

tachycardia, 70, 209, 210, 217
in anaemia, 236, 246
in cardiac failure, 57, 59, 62
paroxysmal, 63, 73
sinus, 70
therapy for, 75, 95
tachydsrhythmias, 48, 50, 54, 55, 63,
    72–3, 209
therapy, **75–6**
tachypnoea,
and parathyroid disorders, 210
and phaeochromocytoma, 217
and poisons, 258
and respiratory disorders, 12, 17, **25, 26**

Taenia spp, 128
tamponade, cardiac, 52, 60, 61
tapeworms, **128, 129**
temperament change, 225
temperature, rectal, 242, 243
in thoracic disease, 31
see also Pyrexia; hypothermia
temporal atrophy, 114, 213
myositis, 114
tenesmus,
differential diagnosis, **189–91**
faecal, 132, 136, 177, 178, **189**
genital, 190
investigation, **190–91**
urinary, 170, 172, 177, 178, 179,
    189–90
Terriers, 213, 218
testicular atrophy, 207, 213
neoplasia, 178, 179, 194, 215
torsion, 122, 242
see also Sertoli cell tumour
tetanus, 66, 114
tetany, lactation, *see* Eclampsia
tetralogy of Fallot, 45, 88
surgery, 92
T wave (ECG), depressed, 54
peaked (spiked), 54, 216
thirst, abnormal, *see* Polydipsia
thoracentesis, 18, 19, **40–42**, 92
thoracic adhesions, 17
capacity, reduced, **26**
duct, erosion, 16
surgery, 20
lavage, 19
neoplasia, 2, 16, 17, 18, 28
percussion, 17, 18, 23, **31**, 79
radiography, 11, 12, **33–4**, 84
radiology, **33–7**
trauma, 16, **22–4**
see also Pleural disorders
thoracotomy, 13, 19, 20, **42**
thorax, penetration, 16, 22
thrill, precordial, 48, 79
thrombasthenia, 238, 245
thrombocythaemia, 238, 245
thrombocytopenia, 228, 238, **245**
in anaemia, 250
autoimmune, **237**, 238, 239
diagnosis, **254**
thromboplastin time, partial, 255
thrombosis, 65
thymic lymphosarcoma, 2, 18
thymoma, 18, 19
thyroid, biopsy, 208, 210
disorders, **206–10**

thyroid, (cont.)
  hormone levels, 207, 208
  neoplasms, 1, 207, 209
  treatment, 208
thyroiditis, lymphocytic, 206, 239
tissue necrosis, 241
tocainide, 73, 76
tomography, radiographic, 37
tonsillitis, 1, 6, 113, 114
tonsils, enlargement, 1
  examination, 2, 3
  neoplasia, 1, 114
toxaemias,
  and acute abdominal disorders, 122
  in anaemia, 247
  in diabetes mellitus, 218
  and diarrhoea, 135
  effect on heart, 51, 58, 70, 99
  hepatic, 147
  in pyometra, 228
  in renal failure, 164, 165–7
  and the stomach, 105, 107
  and vomiting, 112, 113, 117, 119
  in weight loss, 233
toxic drugs, 51, 152
  see also Iatrogenic
toxicity, glycoside, 51, 95, 105
toxoplasmosis, 10, 13, 145, 241
trachea, see also Airway
tracheal
  collapse, 1, 2, 3, 4, 5, 25, 27, 28,
    36, 38
  disorders, 1–2, 5
  hypoplasia, 2
  mucosa, in bronchoscopy, 3, 39
  neoplasms, 1, 3, 38
  obstruction, 1–2
    surgery, 4
  parasites, 1, 3, 4, 5, 6, 36, 38
  pinch, 6
  radiology, 36
  secretions, 38
  trauma, 1, 2, 4, 22
  washings, 3, 6, 38
tracheitis, 5, 6
tracheobronchitis, 5, 38
tracheoscopy, see Bronchoscopy
tracheotomy, 3, 38
transaminase levels; see ALT; AST
transfusions, blood, see Blood
    transfusions
transudate, (true), 17, 41, 168,
    193
  modified, 16, 41, 61, 147, 192
  pericardial, 52

trauma, 258
  abdominal, 126, 192–3, 197
  airway, 1, 4, 22
  biliary, 145, 192, 193
  and blood transfusions, 252
  cardiac, 22, 50, 52, 58
  CNS, in incontinence, 186
    in pulmonary oedema, 10, 23
  intestinal, 126, 192, 241
  pelvic,
    in constipation, 189
    in incontinence, 186
  pulmonary, 10, 14, 22
  renal, 163
  spinal, in collapse, 66
    in incontinence, 186
  thoracic, 16, 22–4
  to urinary tract, 175, 190, 193
travel sickness, 112
trembling, see Muscle tremors
Trichuris vulpis, 128, 131, 133, 135
tricuspid valve, dysplasia, 46, 60
  endocardiosis, 49, 60
  incompetence, 60
trigeminal paralysis, 114
trypsin digest test, 137
  trypsin—like immunoreactivity, 138
TSH stimulation test, 208
tuberculosis, 10, 13, 16, 52, 192, 241
tumour, see neoplasia
tympany, abdominal, 194

ulcer, duodenal, 129
  gastric, 107, 118, 119
  peptic, 192
Uncinaria stenocephala, 128, 135
urachus, pervious, 170, 185
uraemia, 51, 66, 105, 107, 113, 135,
    165, 168, 216, 228
urea,
  level, 123, 147, 151, 164, 166, 168,
    175
ureter, ectopic, 170, 185, 200
  ruptured, 175
urethography, 173, 200
ureterocele, 170, 185, 187
urethral calculus, 183, 184,
  neoplasia, 184
urethritis, 170, 183, 189, 201
urinary calculi, 110, 172
  treatment, 173–4
  catheterization, 122, 171, 173, 174,
    178, 180, 187, 191, 200

urinary calculi, (*cont.*)
for haematuria, 184
for tenesmus, 191
congenital lesions, **170**
haemorrhage, *see* Haematuria
incontinence, *see* Incontinence, urinary
infections, 170, 177, 182, 214, 218, 243
treatment, **171**
obstruction, 122, 163, **172**, 178, 185, 193
surgery, 173, 178
radiology, 171, 173, 174, 175, 184, 187, 197, **199–200**
tenesmus, 170, 172, 177, 178, 179, **189–90**
investigation, **190–91**
tract adhesions, 185
neoplasia, 185, 190
rupture, 192
trauma, **175**, 190, 193
urinalysis, 122, 164, 166, 168, **171, 173**, 178, 228, **231**
in pyrexia, 243
urination, frequency, 170
urine,
acidification, 172, 173
biurate crystals, 151
casts, 164, 168, 228
concentration, **231**
poor, 122, 166, 205, 213, 228
high, 122, 123, 216, 218
culture, **171**, 173, 184
osmolality, **232**
protein content, 168
retention, 174
sample, *see* Urinalysis
s.g., 164, 166, 205, **231**
see also Haematuria; Oliguria
urography, 174, **184**, 187, 191, **200**
uterine disorders, **227–8**
enlargement, **193**, 196, **228**
effect on breathing, 26
effect on heart, 62
rupture, 192
stump adhesions, 185, 190, 201
see also Parturition; Pregnancy; Pyometra

vaccination, for respiratory disease, 6, 29
vagal hyperactivity, 65, 74
excessive, 71
therapy, **74**
tone, 55

vaginal discharge, 183, 184, 228
examination, 183, 187, **191**, 200
polyp, 174, 183, 186, 200
vagino-urethography, 187, **200**
valvular disease, acquired, **49–50**
fibrosis, 49
incompetence, **49**, 58
lesions, congenital, **46**
motion, 89
sites for murmurs, **47**
Van den Bergh test, 150, 156
vascular occlusion, in collapse, 65
in renal failure, 163
resistance, peripheral, 62, 77, 94
ring strictures, 46, 102, 119
surgery for, 92, 103
vasculitis, **246**
vasoconstriction, peripheral, 57
vasodilatation, peripheral, 91, 94
vasodilator therapy, 62, 91, 94, 97
vasomotor tone, reduced, 62, 94
vasovagal syncope, 65
see also Vagal hyperactivity
vena cava, caudal (obstruction), 16, 52, **62**, 148, 193
enlargement, 84, 86, 87
venous congestion, 52, 60, 148
treatment for, 93
obstruction, 16, 52, 62, 64, 148, 193
oxygen level, 60, 88, 89
pressure, central, 123
raised, 60, 61, 62, 88
return, 57
reduced, **62**
ventilatory disorders, **26**, 65
ventricular arrest/standstill, 72, **99**
treatment for, **100**
ectopic beats, **72**, 75
escape rhythm, 70, **72**
failure (left), 62
fibrillation, 74, 75, 99
treatment, 75, **100**
filling (reduced), 62
outflow obstruction, 62
premature beats, **72–3**, 75
septal defect, 45, 61, 88
tachycardias, paroxysmal, **73**, 75
volume overload, 89, 94
vesicular sounds, 11, **32**
vestibular lesions, 111, 112
villous atrophy, **127**, 135, 140
viral hepatitis, *see* Hepatitis, viral
vitamin B deficiency and anaemia, 248
B therapy, 122, 123, 142, 152, 165, 168, 252

vitamin B (*cont.*)
  B$_{12}$ levels, in malabsorption, 138
  D excess, 210, 212, 233
  K therapy, 152, 246, 251, 255, 260
volume
  circulating, 57, 83
  overload, **57**, 61, 88, 89
volvulus, 113, 121
vomiting, **110–13**, 145, 160, 164, 165,
    211, 216, 228
  acute, 113, **121–4**, 125
  differential diagnosis, 113, **121–2**
  in gastric disorders, 106, 107, **113**,
    118, 119
  investigation, **116–20**
  management, 122–4
  persistent, 113, 116–20, 197, 233
  in poisoning, 12, 258
  psychogenic, 112, 119
  radiology, **197**
  stimuli, 111
  in weight loss, 233
vomitus, character, 110, 116
vulva, swollen, 226, 227

weakness, in anaemia, 236, 237, 246, 250
  cardiac, 47, 51, 53, 54, 62, **63**, 74
  differential diagnosis, **65–9**
  endocrine, 207, 210, 211, 213, 216,
    217, 221
  iatrogenic, 94
  neurogenic, 66
weight loss, 11, 12, 17, 30, 50, 61, 119,
    127, 128, 136, 147, 161, 194
  differential diagnosis, **233**
  in endocrine disorders, 205, 209, 211
  investigation, 213, 216, 217, 218, **234**
  in renal failure, 165, 167
West Highland white terriers, 11, 29
Wheaten terrier, 165
whipworms, 128
'wobbler' syndrome, 66, 210
wounds, infected, 241

xanthine derivatives, in therapy, 4, 14,
    96
xylose absorption test, 138, 139

warfarin poisoning, *see* Poisoning,
    warfarin
water consumption, 229, 231
  deprivation test, 205, 213, **231**
'water-hammer' pulse, 78

Yorkshire terriers, 1, 29

zinc therapy, 152